Contemporary Issues in Infectious Disease: Implications for Practice

Editor

JEFFREY KWONG

NURSING CLINICS OF NORTH AMERICA

www.nursing.theclinics.com

Consulting Editor
BENJAMIN SMALLHEER

September 2025 • Volume 60 • Number 3

ELSEVIER

1600 John F. Kennedy Boulevard • Suite 1800 • Philadelphia, Pennsylvania, 19103-2899

http://www.theclinics.com

NURSING CLINICS OF NORTH AMERICA Volume 60, Number 3
September 2025 ISSN 0029-6465, ISBN-13: 978-0-443-29710-6

Editor: Kerry Holland
Developmental Editor: Pallavi Shukla

Publishing Office: *Nursing Clinics of North America* (ISSN 0029-6465) is published bimonthly by Elsevier Inc., 1600 John F. Kennedy Boulevard, Suite 1600, Philadelphia, PA 19103, United States. Periodicals postage paid at New York, NY and additional mailing offices. **USA POSTMASTER**: Send address changes to *Nursing Clinics of North America*, Elsevier Customer Service Department, 3251 Riverport Lane, Maryland Heights, MO 63043, USA. Months of issue are March, June, September, and December. Subscription price per year is, $168.00 (US individuals), $275.00 (international individuals), $231.00 (Canadian individuals), $100.00 (US and Canadian students), and $135.00 (international students). For institutional access pricing please contact Customer Service via the contact information below. To receive student/resident rate, orders must be accompanied by name of affiliated institution, date of term, and the signature of program/residency coordinator on institution letterhead. Orders will be billed at individual rate until proof of status is received. Foreign air speed delivery is included in all *Clinics* subscription prices. All prices are subject to change without notice. Orders, claims, and journal inquiries: Please visit our Support Hub page https://service.elsevier.com for assistance.

Nursing Clinics of North America is covered in *EMBASE/Excerpta Medica, MEDLINE/PubMed (Index Medicus), Social Sciences Citation Index, Current Contents, ASCA, Cumulative Index to Nursing, RNdex Top 100,* and Allied Health Literature and International Nursing Index (INI).

Contributors

CONSULTING EDITOR

BENJAMIN SMALLHEER, PhD, RN, ACNP-BC, FNP-BC, CCRN, CNE, FAANP
Assistant Dean, Master of Science in Nursing Program, Associate Professor, Duke
University School of Nursing, Durham, North Carolina

EDITOR

JEFFREY KWONG, DNP, MPH, AGPCNP-BC, FAANP, FAAN
Currently, Nurse Practitioner, NYU Langone Penn District, New York, New York; Formerly,
Professor, Division of Advanced Nursing Practice, Rutgers, The State University of New
Jersey, Newark, New Jersey

AUTHORS

**AMITA AVADHANI, PhD, DNP, NEA-BC, CNE, DCC, ACNP-BC, AGNP-C, CCRN,
FAANP, FCCM, FNAP**
Chair and Professor, Department of Nursing, College of Public Health, Temple University,
Philadelphia, Pennsylvania

ALANNA BERGMAN, PhD, AGNP-BC, RN
Post Doctoral Fellow, School of Nursing, University of Virginia, Charlottesville, Virginia

SHERILYN CAMILLE BRINKLEY, BA, BSN, MSN, NP
Nurse Practitioner Manager, Division of Infectious Diseases, Johns Hopkins University,
Fisher Center, Baltimore, Maryland

COURTNEY BROWN, MSN, ANP-BC
Graduate Nursing Faculty, School of Nursing and Public Health, Moravian University,
Bethlehem, Pennsylvania

MARY DIGIULIO, DNP, ANP-BC, GNP-BC, FAANP
Director DNP Program, Director CRNP Programs, School of Nursing and Public Health,
Moravian University, Bethlehem, Pennsylvania

SUSAN DOYLE-LINDRUD, DNP, APN
Professor of Nursing, Columbia University School of Nursing, New York, New York

COURTNEY DUBOIS SHIHABUDDIN, DNP, APRN-CNP, AGPCNP-BC
Assistant Clinical Professor, Specialty Track Director, Adult-Gerontology Primary Care
Nurse Practitioner Program, Specialty Track Director, Adult-Gerontology Clinical Nurse
Specialist Program, Medical Director of Quality, The Columbus Free Clinic, The Ohio State
University-College of Nursing, Columbus, Ohio

CHRISTOPHER GLEASON, MSN, FNP-C
United States Army Reserve Captain, Family Nurse Practitioner, Primary Care, Veterans
Health Administration; Unites States Army Reserve, Montana, Virginia

JASON GLEASON, DNP, FNP-C, FAANP
USAF Lieutenant Colonel (RET), Nurse Practitioner, Primary Care, Veterans Health Administration, Montana, Virginia; Faculty Member, Fitzgerald Health Education Associates By Colilbri, Lawrence, Massachusetts

JOELLE D. HARGRAVES, DNP, MSN, RN, CCRN, CCNS
Associate Professor of Instruction (Nursing), College of Public Health, Temple University, Philadelphia, Pennsylvania

MATT F. HOFFMAN, DNP, APRN, FNP-C
Clinical Associate Professor, School of Nursing, Assistant Dean, Round Rock College of Nursing, Texas A&M University, Round Rock, Texas

RYAN HOLLEY-MALLO, PhD, DNP, NP-C, FAANP
Associate Professor of Graduate Nursing, Beal University, Bangor, Maine; Nurse Practitioner, Department of Family and Emergency Medicine, Sheridan Community Hospital, Sheridan, Michigan

MARY KOSLAP-PETRACO, DNP, PPCNP-BC, CPNP, FAANP
Clinical Assistant Professor, Stony Brook University, School of Nursing, Nurse Consultant, Immunize.org, CEO/Owner, Pediatric Nurse Practitioner House Calls, Massapequa Park, New York

JEFFREY KWONG, DNP, MPH, AGPCNP-BC, FAANP, FAAN
Currently, Nurse Practitioner, NYU Langone Penn District, New York, New York; Formerly, Professor, Division of Advanced Nursing Practice, Rutgers, The State University of New Jersey, Newark, New Jersey

GABRIEL LEE, BS
Medical Student, College of Medicine, The Ohio State University, Columbus, Ohio

MICHAEL McINTOSH, PhD, RN, CIC
Manager Infection Prevention - Ambulatory, Cooper University Health Care, Camden, New Jersey

CLARE CARDO McKEGNEY, DNP, CPNP-PC
Associate Professor, Columbia University, School of Nursing, New York City, New York

TERI MOSER WOO, PhD, ARNP, CPNP-PC, FAANP
Pediatric ARNP, Mary Bridge Children's Pediatric Urgent Care, Puyallup, Washington; Professor and Director of HRSA Nursing Workforce Diversity Grant, Saint Martin's University, Lacey, Washington

ANGELA OTTO-RYAN, DNP, CPNP-PC, CBC
Instructor, Division of Entry to Baccalaureate Practice, Rutgers Health School of Nursing, Newark, New Jersey

MARGARET QUINN, DNP, CPNP-PC, CPNP, CNE
Clinical Professor, Rutgers Health School of Nursing, Newark, New Jersey

BERNADETTE SHEERON, DNP, AGACNP-BC, ANP-BC
Assistant Professor of Instruction (Nursing), College of Public Health, Temple University, Philadelphia, Pennsylvania

TANIA THOMAS, MD, MPH
Associate Professor, Division of Infectious Diseases and International Health, University of Virginia School of Medicine, University of Virginia, Charlottesville, Virginia

DANIEL P. WORRALL, MSN, ANP-BC
Nurse Practitioner, Massachusetts General Hospital, Sexual Health Clinic, Boston, Massachusetts

Contents

Pneumococci are the most common bacterial cause of childhood pneumonia, especially in children aged younger than 5 years. In adults, pneumococci account for 10% to 30% of adult community-acquired pneumonia. The conjugate pneumococcal vaccines have been shown to have a remarkable effect, reducing the incidence of all types of pneumococcal diseases. Overtime the vaccines have been updated to include protection against more serotypes. Schedules for administration have also changed based on age and pre-existing conditions. Development and implementation of pneumococcal vaccines and racial disparities are discussed.

Respiratory syncytial virus (RSV) is a leading viral cause of respiratory infections in young children, especially affecting infants aged under 6 months, preterm infants, and those with underlying health conditions. It can result in bronchiolitis, pneumonia, and respiratory failure. Recent advancements in RSV prevention, particularly maternal vaccination and monoclonal antibodies for infants, show promise in reducing the global impact of the disease. This article provides an overview of RSV, with a focus on current preventive strategies and the significant breakthroughs that aim to lessen its burden on vulnerable populations.

Measles is a highly transmissible viral disease that is preventable through vaccination. Despite global initiatives, outbreaks persist, demonstrating the need for high immunization coverage. Spread occurs via respiratory droplets and airborne particles, reinforcing the need for herd immunity. Symptoms include fever, cough, and a distinctive rash. Complications may include pneumonia, encephalitis, and in rare cases, acute disseminated encephalomyelitis and subacute sclerosing panencephalitis. Diagnosis relies on reverse transcription-polymerase chain reaction and serology tests. Two doses of the measles, mumps, and rubella vaccine remains the most effective preventive measure and is essential for controlling and eliminating measles outbreaks.

Tick-borne infections are a growing public health concern in North America. Geographic areas of tick populations are expanding and may be impacted by climate change, animal migration, urbanization, or deforestation. Tick-borne infections are challenging to diagnose due to their nonspecific symptoms and many people do not recall a specific tick bite. The true incidence of tick-borne infections is unknown as there are asymptomatic patients and case identification and reporting requirements vary geographically. Early identification and treatment is critical for recovery and, in some cases, prevention of death or long-term complications.

Norovirus is one of the leading causes of infectious gastroenteritis globally, with over 685 million cases occurring annually. This highly infectious enteric pathogen can lead to dehydration and severe illness, especially in pediatric patients, older adults, and those who are immunocompromised. Transmission and spread of norovirus often lead to regional outbreaks across the United States each year. Early symptom recognition and implementation of prevention strategies can reduce the spread of this infection. This article provides an overview of the epidemiology, pathogenesis, clinical presentation, management, and prevention recommendations for norovirus. The role of nurses is also highlighted.

Prescribing antibiotics in a time of increasing resistance requires the prescriber to understand the mechanisms of how pathogens develop resistance, pathogens that are of the highest concern to impact health outcomes, and guidelines for first-line treatment for infections. It is important to know antimicrobial resistance patterns and utilize a local antibiogram when prescribing to treat an infection empirically. Case study examples of using national guidelines and local antibiograms to provide optimal care are discussed.

Incidence of hospital-acquired infections (HAIs) has increased after the pandemic leading to worsening health outcomes, especially in vulnerable populations including elderly patients. Simple practices such as effective handwashing can help mitigate HAI incidence. Hospitals and health care workers must do more to minimize the risks of HAIs.

Susan Doyle-Lindrud

Neutropenic fever is a medical emergency that requires prompt evaluation. Neutropenic fever is defined as a single oral temperature $\geq$ 38.3°C (101.0°F) or a sustained temperature $\geq$ 38.0°C (101.0°F) for 1 hour and an absolute neutrophil count of less than 0.5×10^9/L. The management of these patients includes initiation of broad-spectrum antibiotic within 1 hour of presentation. Lab work and blood cultures should be obtained prior to starting antibiotics and patients should be assessed for risk of serious complications of febrile neutropenia utilizing the Multinational Association of Supportive Care in Cancer or Clinical Index of Stable Febrile Neutropenia scoring system.

Alanna Bergman and Tania Thomas

Tuberculosis (TB) remains an ongoing threat. TB requires exposure to *Mycobacterium tuberculosis*, but disease development is driven by exposure, infectiousness, susceptibility, and environment. TB elimination requires increased awareness about TB prevention and treatment strategies. The centers of TB excellence complement current guidelines from the Center for Disease Control and Prevention, the National TB Coalition of America, and the Infectious Disease Society of America to support nurses and providers. Enhanced contact investigation, prevention, and treatment will aid in the pathway to a TB-free North America. To address disparities in TB, nurses in practice, research, and policy settings must address individual, interpersonal, and organizational barriers to care and ongoing treatment adherence.

Sherilyn Camille Brinkley

Hepatitis C is a chronic, life-threatening liver disease on the rise in the United States primarily among young adults. Despite the availability of highly effective, well-tolerated, and easy to use treatments, roughly half of those living with HCV remain undiagnosed and less than one-third of those diagnosed receive timely treatment. There are multiple patient, provider, and systemic barriers to care requiring a well-funded, multi-pronged approach to overcome obstacles along the HCV care continuum to advance elimination goals.

Daniel P. Worrall

Cases of syphilis in the United States are at an all-time high. Although men who have sex with men continue to be adversely affected, record rates of infection are now seen in women, men who have sex with women, and in congenital cases. Persons of color and ethnic minorities are among communities affected. Review of sexual practices and risk factors such as substance use are key to identifying infections early to stop spread of the disease. Educating nurses on how to identify those at risk, order and interpret testing, effectively treat, and follow these patients is vital to stopping the epidemic.

Current Challenges in Gonorrhea Management: A Focus on Diagnosis, Treatment, and Antimicrobial Resistance

Gabriel Lee, Matt F. Hoffman, and Courtney DuBois Shihabuddin

Gonorrhea, caused by *Neisseria gonorrhoeae*, remains the second most common bacterial sexually transmitted infection in the United States, with approximately 1.57 million new infections annually. The growing challenge of antimicrobial resistance (AMR) in *N gonorrhoeae* has led to critical screening and treatment guidelines advancements. This study provides a comprehensive review of gonorrhea's epidemiology, pathophysiology, and clinical manifestations. The study also highlights the role of expedited partner therapy and the need for enhanced patient education to prevent reinfection. The discussion emphasizes the importance of ongoing surveillance, updated clinical practices, and health education to combat the rising rates of gonorrhea and the spread of AMR.

Diagnosis and Management of Bacterial Prostatitis

Ryan Holley-Mallo, Jason Gleason, and Christopher Gleason

Prostatitis remains one of the number one reasons for primary and urologic care visits annually for men across the lifespan. Most cases of acute bacterial prostatitis are attributed to Escherichia coli with a smaller number of cases being attributed to sexually transmitted infections and are easily treatable in the outpatient setting. However, cases of chronic prostatitis often require a team-based approach-to-care and both pharmaceutical and non-pharmaceutical interventions. New and investigative treatments are currently being studied for their role in the treatment and management of chronic prostatitis, but additional studies are needed to determine their efficacy.

NURSING CLINICS

SERIES OF RELATED INTEREST

Advances in Family Practice Nursing
www.advancesinfamilypracticenursing.com

THE CLINICS ARE AVAILABLE ONLINE!
Access your subscription at:
www.theclinics.com

Foreword

The Changing Landscape of Infectious Disease Management

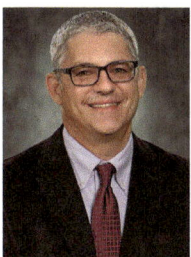

Benjamin Smallheer, PhD, RN, ACNP-BC, FNP-BC, CCRN, CNE, FAANP
Consulting Editor

The scope of infectious disease care spans all body systems, health care settings, and clinical roles, creating a complex landscape of evolving pathogens, therapeutic advancements, and emerging threats. Among these, viral infections remain a critical focus, affecting gastrointestinal, respiratory, and hepatic infections.

Foodborne illness outbreaks continue to pose significant public health challenges, leading to thousands of illnesses, hundreds of hospitalizations, and multiple fatalities. According to the US Centers for Disease Control and Prevention (CDC), an estimated 48 million, or one in six, experience foodborne illness annually, with 128,000 hospitalizations and 3000 deaths reported each year.[1] Digestive system diseases account for 8.4 million emergency department visits, with Norovirus recognized as a leading cause of foodborne illness. Other pathogens, including Salmonella, Shiga toxin-producing E coli, and Campylobacter, significantly contribute to these statistics.[2]

As viruses evolve, so does our understanding of their mechanisms, diagnostic trends, therapeutic options, and prevention strategies. Advancements in genomic sequencing technologies have increased the ability to identify and track pathogens rapidly, leading to more responsive treatment protocols and accelerated vaccine development, such as those targeting measles-rubella. Notably, the CDC's initiatives have contributed to higher viral load suppression rates among children living with HIV, demonstrating the impact of coordinated public health efforts.

Antibiotic stewardship remains fundamental to bacterial infection management, requiring a multidisciplinary approach to balance effective treatment with the growing challenge of antimicrobial resistance. The use of antibiograms, alongside rigorous considerations of drug-resistant organisms, is essential in guiding appropriate antimicrobial therapy. Immunosuppressed patients, particularly those presenting with neutropenic fever, demand swift, evidence-based interventions to prevent severe complications.

Nurs Clin N Am 60 (2025) xiii–xiv
https://doi.org/10.1016/j.cnur.2025.06.001
0029-6465/25/© 2025 Published by Elsevier Inc.

Sexually transmitted infections (STIs) also represent a key domain where advancements in diagnostics and treatment have strengthened patient care and reduced long-term complications. Modern approaches prioritize both preventive and therapeutic measures, reshaping the landscape of STI health care delivery.

In addition, atypical and persistent infections—such as rare bacterial, fungal, and parasitic diseases—warrant ongoing clinical vigilance. Though often overlooked, these conditions require comprehensive medical awareness to ensure optimal patient outcomes.

This issue of *Nursing Clinics of North America* brings together expert perspectives, evidence-based practices, and the latest clinical insights to support infectious disease clinicians and nursing professionals alike. By addressing these pressing topics, we contribute to the evolving understanding of infectious disease medicine, equipping health care providers with the knowledge and strategies necessary to improve patient care in an ever-changing health care landscape.

Benjamin Smallheer, PhD, RN, ACNP-BC, FNP-BC, CCRN, CNE, FAANP
Duke University School of Nursing
307 Trent Drive
Box 3322, Office 3117
Durham, NC 27710, USA

E-mail address:
benjamin.smallheer@duke.edu

REFERENCES

1. Center for Disease Control and Prevention. About food safety. U.S. Department of Health and Human Services. 2024. Available at: https://www.cdc.gov/food-safety/about/index.html. Accessed June 3, 2025.
2. Center for Disease Control and Prevention. FastStats: digestive diseases. National Center for Health Statistics. 2023. Available at: https://www.cdc.gov/nchs/fastats/digestive-diseases.htm. Accessed June 3, 2025.

Preface

Infectious and Emerging Diseases Special Issue

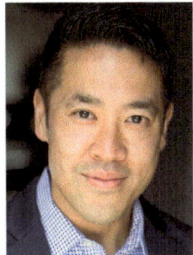

Jeffrey Kwong, DNP, MPH, AGPCNP-BC
Editor

According to the Centers for Disease Control and Prevention's National Center for Health Statistics,[1] infectious or parasitic diseases are associated with 10.2 million outpatient office visits, 3.8 million emergency department visits, and 482,000 hospital admissions annually. Needless to say, in 2020, the world experienced the impact and devastation of a global infectious disease outbreak with the spread of SARS-CoV-2 (COVID-19). The lingering effects of the COVID-19 pandemic can still be experienced to this day.

Although there were many lessons learned from COVID-19, it is important to realize that there are numerous other infections that are associated with morbidity and mortality. Furthermore, new and emerging infectious diseases have the potential to pose a threat to the health of our nation and our public health infrastructure. With the increase in infectious diseases in the United States and globally, there has been a growing focus on the rise of antibiotic resistance, opportunities for prevention of infections, as well as issues of health equity in the context of access to care and immunizations. I was honored when I was asked to help edit and curate the articles for this special issue. This issue of *Nursing Clinics of North America* highlights some of the emerging topics in the field of infectious disease, provides a review of common infections seen in the acute care and ambulatory settings, and highlights the latest information on prevention of emerging and re-emerging infections for patients across the life span. Nurses in all settings play a vital role in identifying, assessing, treating, and

Nurs Clin N Am 60 (2025) xv–xvi
https://doi.org/10.1016/j.cnur.2024.11.001
0029-6465/25/© 2024 Published by Elsevier Inc.

nursing.theclinics.com

preventing infectious diseases. I hope that you find the information in this issue beneficial for your clinical practice.

Jeffrey Kwong, DNP, MPH, AGPCNP-BC
Currently, Nurse Practitioner
NYU Langone Penn District
New York, NY, USA

Formerly, Professor
Division of Advanced Nursing Practice, Rutgers
The State University of New Jersey
Newark, NJ, USA

E-mail address:
Jeffrey.Kwong@nyulangone.org

REFERENCE

1. Centers for Disease Control and Prevention. National Center for Health Statistics, Infectious Disease. Available at: https://www.cdc.gov/nchs/fastats/infectious-disease.htm (Accessed 12 November 2024).

Pneumococcal Vaccine

Mary Koslap-Petraco, DNP, PPCNP-BC, CPNP

KEYWORDS

- *Streptococcus pneumoniae* • Pneumococci • Vaccines • Racial disparities
- Vaccine administration • Vaccine schedules

KEY POINTS

- Pneumococci are the most common bacterial cause of childhood pneumonia, especially in children aged younger than 5 years.
- Pneumococcal infections cause a plethora of illness across the life span, but they particularly affect the very young and the very old.
- Pneumococcal vaccines have been available for years and updated formulations offer more opportunities to provide protection to individuals over a range of ages and conditions.

INTRODUCTION

There cannot be a discussion of pneumococcal vaccine without first reviewing the diseases that the vaccine prevents and the impact of these infections on the population. *Streptococcus pneumoniae* causes acute bacterial infections. The bacterium, also called pneumococcus, was first isolated by Louis Pasteur in 1881 from the saliva of a patient with rabies.[1] The association between pneumococcus and lobar pneumonia was first described in 1883, but pneumococcal pneumonia was confused with other types of pneumonia until the development of the Gram stain in 1884. Between 1915 and 1945, the chemical structure and antigenicity of the pneumococcal capsular polysaccharide (CPS), its association with virulence, and the role of bacterial polysaccharides in human disease were described. More than 80 serotypes of pneumococci had been described by 1940.[1]

Efforts to develop effective pneumococcal vaccines began as early as 1911. However, with the advent of penicillin in the 1940s, interest in pneumococcal vaccination declined until it was observed that many patients still died despite antibiotic treatment.[1] By the late 1960s, efforts were again being made to develop a polyvalent pneumococcal vaccine. The first pneumococcal vaccine was licensed for use in the United States in 1977. The first conjugate pneumococcal vaccine was licensed in the United States in 2000.[1]

Stony Brook University School of Nursing, 101 Nicolls Road, Stony Brook, NY 11794-8240, USA
E-mail addresses: mary.koslap-petraco@stonybrook.edu; petraconp@gmail.com

Nurs Clin N Am 60 (2025) 399–410
https://doi.org/10.1016/j.cnur.2024.10.003
0029-6465/25/© 2024 Elsevier Inc. All rights reserved, including those for text and data mining, AI training, and similar technologies.

nursing.theclinics.com

Description of Streptococcus pneumoniae

S pneumoniae bacteria are lancet-shaped, gram-positive, facultative anaerobic organisms. They are typically observed in pairs (diplococci) but may also occur singularly or in short chains. Most pneumococci are encapsulated, and their surfaces are composed of complex polysaccharides. Polysaccharide capsules determine pathogenicity, antigenicity, and serotype. Type-specific antibody to CPS is protective against disease caused by that serotype. One hundred serotypes were documented as of 2020, based on their reaction with type-specific antisera. Serotype prevalence differs by age and geographic area.[1]

Morbidity and Mortality of Pneumococcal Disease in Adults and Children

The clinical spectrum of pneumococcal infections ranges from invasive disease with infection of normally sterile sites that include osteomyelitis, bacteremia without a focus of infection, pneumonia with bacteremia, septic arthritis, and meningitis to noninvasive infections such as pneumonia without bacteremia, otitis media, and sinusitis.[1] Group B Streptococcus is a common cause of bacterial meningitis in infants aged less than 2 months. The mortality rate from meningitis is 8% in children and 22% in adults, and long-term neurologic complications are reported in 50% of survivors. S pneumoniae is the most common cause in all other age groups, with the exception of 11 to 17 year olds, where Neisseria meningitidis is still the most common cause.[2] Pneumonia is the most common illness caused by S pneumoniae in the United States in adults. There are over 150,000 hospitalizations from pneumococcal pneumonia, and they are often complications of influenza. The mortality rate is 5% to 7%, with higher rates in older adults. Pneumococcal bacteremia is responsible for approximately 20% mortality rate, with up to 60% mortality in older adults.[3] Annually there are 7500 to more than 10,500 deaths caused by pneumococcal pneumonia, and more that 3000 deaths due to pneumococcal meningitis and bacteremia.[3]

Pneumococci are the most common bacterial cause of childhood pneumonia, especially in children aged younger than 5 years. Pneumococci are a common cause of acute otitis media in children. In adults, pneumococci account for 10% to 30% of adult community-acquired pneumonia.[1] Before the routine use of pneumococcal conjugate vaccine (PCV), the annual burden in children aged younger than 5 years was a significant 17,000 cases of invasive disease, 200 deaths from invasive pneumococcal disease (IPD), and 5 million cases of acute otitis media.[4]

In the United States, prior to the widespread use of a 7 valent pneumococcal conjugate vaccine (PCV7), the 7 most common serotypes isolated from blood or cerebrospinal fluid (CSF) of children aged younger than 5 years accounted for 80% of infections. Additionally, these 7 serotypes accounted for about 50% of isolates from older children and adults.[5] Since the introduction of a 13 valent pneumococcal conjugate vaccine (PCV13), invasive disease caused by PCV13 serotypes declined by 90% in children.[6]

Epidemiology and Streptococcus pneumoniae Colonization

Pneumococci commonly inhabit the respiratory tract, and rates of asymptomatic colonization in healthy adults are highly variable (5%–90%) and depend on several factors, including age and environment. Among school-age children, 20% to 60% may be colonized. Only 5% to 10% of adults without children are colonized; however, on military installations, as many as 50% to 60% of service personnel may be colonized. The duration of carriage varies and is generally longer in children than in adults. The relationship of carriage to the development of natural immunity is poorly understood.[1]

Risk Factors for Streptococcus pneumoniae Colonization

Several factors can influence the risk for pneumococcal infections including severe infections. These risk factors can be different between children and adults (**Boxes 1–3**).[3]

Racial Disparities in Pneumococcal Disease Outcomes

Compared with adults of other races and ethnicities, Black adults with IPD tend to have significantly worse outcomes.[7] Black adults experience up to 12% higher prevalence of nonimmunocompromising high-risk conditions over other ethnic groups putting these Black adults at greater risk for pneumococcal infections. This high-risk group also experienced longer hospital stays and higher hospitalization costs than other than non-Blacks in all age and discharge status groups for nonbacteremic pneumonia and for Blacks discharged alive with IPD. Costs were higher for Blacks aged 65 years or older with IPD. The rates of age-specific mortality due to IPD are 1% to 12% higher in Blacks.[7] Introduction of PCV13 was associated with substantial reductions in overall incidence and socioeconomic and racial disparities in PCV13-serotype incidence. The introduction of pneumococcal vaccines has helped to reduce—but not eliminate—racial disparities in IPD incidence.[8]

Antibiotic Resistance and Streptococcus pneumoniae

Pneumococcal bacteria that cause IPD are resistant to one or more classes of antibiotics in more than 40% of cases. S pneumoniae resistant to at least one antibiotic causes more than 2 in 5 infections. The proportion of IPD not susceptible to select antibiotics has remained relatively steady over time. New pneumococcal vaccines will be critical as the proportion of resistance to some important antibiotics continues to increase.[9]

Vaccine-Related Serotype Replacement

Serotype replacement occurs when environmental pressures lead to the expansion of certain (often previously rare) serotypes. Nonvaccine serotypes make up an increasing proportion of pneumococcal disease cases. This is particularly common in people with comorbidities and in older adults.[9] Although rates of antimicrobial resistance have decreased overall, antimicrobial-resistant non-PCV13 serotypes have increased in incidence.[10] The emergence of these antimicrobial-resistant serotypes has led to the development of updated pneumococcal vaccines that cover emerging serotypes.

A major concern was the rapid unexpected rise in the serotypes that caused serious disease, serotypes 19A and 3 after the introduction of PCV7. Serotype 19A soon rose to be the most prominent, but it started declining again after the introduction of

---

Box 1
Risk factors in children

- Younger age
- Exposure to cigarette smoke
- Group childcare
- Crowded living conditions
- Presence of young siblings
- Alaska Native, African American, and some American Indian race/ethnicity

Adapted from CDC Pneumococcal Disease.[3]

Box 2
Risk factor in adults

- Current cigarette use
- Regular contact with children
- Nonurban geographic location
- Nursing home residence
- Alcoholism
- CSF leak
- Chronic heart, kidney, liver, or lung disease
- Cochlear implant
- Decreased immune function from disease or drugs (ie, immunocompromising condition)
- Diabetes mellitus
- Crowded living conditions or homelessness
- Alaska Native, African American, and some American Indian race/ethnicity
- Chronic lung conditions that increase risk include chronic obstructive pulmonary disease, emphysema, and asthma

People with a cochlear implant appear to be at an increased risk for pneumococcal meningitis specifically

Adapted from CDC Pneumococcal Disease.[3]

PCV13, which included this serotype. This serotype is associated not only with strong invasive capacity but also with multiple antibiotic resistance. Throughout carriage studies, serotype 19A not only increased its prevalence from 1.4% in the pre-PCV era to 11.5% within 3 years but also accounted for a significant proportion of both penicillin-nonsusceptibility and macrolide resistance in the latter period (36.3% and 52.1%, respectively).[11] The prevalence of serotype 19A decreased back again to 0.5% by 2015 to 2016.[12]

The other serotype that had raised concerns is serotype 3. While, it is almost entirely sensitive to antibiotics, it has high invasive potential and case-fatality rate (>15%). Despite its inclusion in PCV13, it is not only kept its second position among IPDs in

---

Box 3
Immunocompromising conditions that put individuals at an increased risk for pneumococcal infection

Examples of immunocompromising conditions include
- Chronic renal failure or nephrotic syndrome
- Congenital or acquired asplenia or splenic dysfunction
- Congenital or acquired immunodeficiency
- Disease or condition treated with immunosuppressive drugs or radiation therapy[a]
- Human immunodeficiency virus infection
- Sickle cell disease or other hemoglobinopathies

[a]This includes Hodgkin disease, leukemias, lymphomas, malignant neoplasms, and solid organ transplant.

Adapted from CDC Pneumococcal Disease.[3]

Europe but also has increased slightly. Conversely, serotype 3 is seen less in carriage.[10]

While the more recent PCV15, PVC20, and PCV21 have covered an increasing number of serotypes, these still represent only a relatively small proportion of the nearly 100 different capsular serotypes. Pneumococci respond extremely rapidly to the vaccine pressure—increasing vaccine valency continuously, based on the newly emerging serotypes, would lead to an endless battle between the pneumococci and us. Therefore, alternative approaches in vaccine development have also been considered. These include protein-based vaccines, which target antigens that are conserved across all serotypes.[13] Whole-cell vaccines containing either killed[14] or live attenuated bacteria[15] are other approaches being considered. The results of these studies indicate that these vaccines may be able to completely eliminate the pneumococcus even from the nasopharynx.[16]

Conjugated Versus Polysaccharide Chain Vaccines

Conjugate vaccines have been developed to induce a robust immune response against bacterial CPSs. CPSs are long polymers composed of many repeating units of simple sugars and serve as a protective external layer for many bacteria. Depending on the chemical composition of the repeating unit (usually composed of 1–7 monosaccharides). Bacteria can synthesize hundreds of chemically and immunologically different polysaccharides. Antibodies against the polysaccharides of many pathogenic bacteria, such as meningococcus, haemophilus influenzae type b (Hib), and pneumococcus, protect people from disease. Vaccines composed of purified polysaccharides against meningococcus and pneumococcus were developed in the 1970s. Unfortunately, those vaccines, while partially immunogenic in adults, were completely unable to induce an antibody response in infants and children, the population for whom the vaccines were mostly needed. Polysaccharide vaccines are weakly immunogenic and produce antibodies but no T-cell response.[17] This problem was overcome in the 1980s when John Robbins and Rachel Schneerson at the National Institutes of Health in Bethesda, Maryland, and David Smith and Porter Anderson in Rochester, New York, independently noted an interesting phenomenon. They observed that in 1929, it was reported that bacterial CPSs become very immunogenic when covalently linked to a carrier protein.[18] Goebel[19] began work on a conjugate vaccine against Hib, which worked exceptionally well in infants and children. At the same time, conjugate vaccines were developed for meningococcus[20] and pneumococcus,[21] and both were licensed in 1999 and 2000 in the United Kingdom and United States, respectively.

The Pneumococcal polysaccharide vaccine 23 valent (PPV23) contains the purified capsular polysaccharide of 23 different serotypes, and it has been available since the early 1980s. The generation of conjugate vaccines that included 10 (PCV10) or 13 (PCV13) different serotypes, covalently conjugated to strongly immunogenic bacterial carrier proteins. Unlike PPV23, these vaccines have completely changed the pneumococcal epidemiology worldwide, very rapidly after they were licensed and their widespread use began during the early 2000s.[22] The latest updated vaccines are also conjugated vaccines. Conjugated vaccines are much more immunogenic and produce a more robust immune response. Conjugated vaccines also boost immunity much more robustly than polysaccharide vaccines.[23]

The conjugate pneumococcal vaccines have been shown to have a remarkable effect, reducing the incidence of all types of pneumococcal diseases. As the PCVs were developed specifically against pediatric IPDs, the most drastic reductions were observed in IPD among children aged less than 5 years. According to the US-wide

Centers for Disease Control and Prevention (CDC) surveillance data, the overall IPD incidence (ie, number of cases per 100,000 population) in this age category declined from 95 cases in 1998 to 9 cases in 2016. IPD caused by PCV13 serotypes declined from 88 to 2 cases.[24]

Although the PCV-vaccinated individuals were the children, transmission of pneumococci to unvaccinated populations can be prevented by vaccinating the children, thanks to the so-called herd effect. A large-scale US study conducted by Moore and colleagues[22] showed that the overall IPD incidence in adults also declined by 12% to 32%, depending on age. In addition, the reduction of mortality rates was also observed, particularly among patients aged greater than 50 years. They estimated that due to the combined effect of PCV7 and PCV13, nearly 400,000 cases of IPD and about 30,000 deaths had been prevented between 2001 and 2012. Consequently, the recommendation of PCVs was extended to adults as well and suggested the basic schedule, which is a PCV first, later followed by PPV23 for higher serotype coverage.[25]

Introduction of Pneumococcal Vaccines

The first pneumococcal polysaccharide vaccine was licensed for use in the United States in 1977. It contained purified capsular polysaccharide antigen from 14 different types of pneumococci. In 1983, a 23 valent polysaccharide vaccine (pneumococcal Polysaccharide vaccine 23 valent [PPSV23], Pneumovax 23 - Rahway, NJ) was licensed and replaced the 14 valent vaccine, which is no longer produced.[1]

The first PCV (Prevnar 7 - Pennsylvania; Madison, NJ, PCV7) was licensed for use in the United States in 2000. It included purified capsular polysaccharide of 7 serotypes of S pneumoniae. In 2010, a PCV13 (Prevnar 13 - Wyeth) was licensed in the United States. It contains the same 7 serotypes of S pneumoniae as PCV7 plus serotypes 1, 3, 5, 6A, 7F, and 19A.[1]

In 2008, the serotypes covered in PCV13 caused 53%, 49%, and 44% of IPD cases among persons aged 18 through 49 years, 50 through 64 years, and 65 years or older, respectively; serotypes covered in PPSV23 caused 78%, 76%, and 66% of IPD cases among persons in these age groups.[1]

Types and composition of pneumococcal vaccines

Currently licensed pneumococcal conjugate vaccines. PCVs are differentiated by the number of serotypes they protect against.[26]

PCV21 (CAPVAXIVE) is a sterile solution of purified capsular polysaccharides from S pneumoniae serotypes 3, 6A, 7F, 8, 9N, 10A, 11A, 12F, 15A, 15B (de-O-acetylated prior to conjugation), 16F, 17F, 19A, 20A, 22F, 23A, 23B, 24F, 31, 33F, and 35B individually conjugated to cross reacting material non-toxic mutant of diphtheria toxin (non-toic mutant of diphtheria toxin (CRM197) carrier protein. A 0.5 mL PCV21 dose contains a total of 84 mcg of pneumococcal polysaccharide antigen (4 mcg each of polysaccharide serotypes 3, 6A, 7F, 8, 9N, 10A, 11A, 12F, 15A, 15B [deOAc 15B], 16F, 17F, 19A, 20A, 22F, 23A, 23B, 24F, 31, 33F, and 35B) conjugated to approximately 65 mcg of CRM197 carrier protein, 1.55 mg L-histidine, 0.50 mg of polysorbate 20, 4.49 mg sodium chloride, and water for injection. The vaccine does not contain any preservatives.

PCV20 (Prevnar20 - New York, NY) is a sterile suspension of saccharides from 20 serotypes of S pneumoniae (1, 3, 4, 5, 6A, 6B, 7F, 8, 9V, 10A, 11A, 12F, 14, 15B, 18C, 19A, 19F, 22F, 23F, and 33F) individually linked to a nontoxic variant of diphtheria toxin known as CRM197. A 0.5 mL dose contains approximately 2.2 µg of saccharides from each of 19 serotypes, approximately 4.4 µg of saccharides from serotype 6B, 51 µg CRM197 carrier protein, 100 µg polysorbate 80, 295 µg succinate buffer, 4.4 mg sodium chloride, and 125 µg aluminum as aluminum phosphate adjuvant.[26]

PCV15 (Vaxneuvance - Merck) is a sterile suspension of purified capsular polysaccharides from 15 serotypes of *S pneumoniae* (1, 3, 4, 5, 6A, 6B, 7F, 9V, 14, 18C, 19A, 19F, 22F, 23F, and 33F) individually conjugated to a nontoxic variant of diphtheria toxin known as CRM197. A 0.5 mL PCV15 dose contains 2.0 μg of polysaccharide from each of 14 serotypes and 4.0 μg of polysaccharide from serotype 6B, 30 μg of CRM197 carrier protein, 1.55 mg L-histidine, 1 mg of polysorbate 20, 4.50 mg sodium chloride, and 125 μg of aluminum as aluminum phosphate adjuvant. The vaccine does not contain any preservatives.[26]

Currently licensed polysaccharide vaccine. *Pneumococcal polysaccharide vaccine, or PPSV23* (Pneumovax 23), includes purified preparations of pneumococcal capsular polysaccharide. PPSV23 contains polysaccharide antigen from 23 types of pneumococcal bacteria. It contains 25 μg of each antigen per dose and contains 0.25% phenol as a preservative.[26]

Immunogenicity, vaccine efficacy, and safety

Twenty-one valent pneumococcal conjugate vaccine The Food and Drug Administration (FDA) licensed PCV21 in 2024 for use in individuals aged 18 years and older. Studies showed that PCV21-induced antibody levels comparable to PCV15, PCV20, or PPSV23 for the shared serotypes in adults aged 50 years and older. Studies have shown the safety of PCV21 to be comparable to the safety of PCV15, PCV20, and PPSV23.[26]

Fifteen valent pneumococcal conjugate vaccine and 20 valent pneumococcal conjugate vaccine FDA licensed PCV15 and PCV20 in 2021 for use in adults. Studies showed they induced antibody levels comparable to those induced by PCV13 or PPSV23. The studies also showed PCV15 and PCV20 were safe compared with PCV13 with or without PPSV23.

FDA approved PCV15 in 2022 and PCV20 in 2023 for use in children aged 6 weeks through 17 years. This was based on clinical trial data showing they induced antibody levels comparable to those induced by PCV13. The studies also showed that safety of PCV15 and PCV20 were comparable to that of PCV13.[26]

Seven valent pneumococcal conjugate vaccine and 13 valent pneumococcal conjugate vaccine Substantial evidence demonstrates routine infant PCV7 and PCV13 vaccination reduced pneumococcal carriage and transmission of vaccine serotypes. This resulted in lower IPD incidence among unvaccinated persons of all ages, including infants too young to receive the vaccine. Compared to unvaccinated children, children who received PCV7

- Had 20% fewer episodes of chest radiograph-confirmed pneumonia
- Had 7% fewer episodes of acute otitis media
- Underwent 20% fewer tympanostomy tube placements[26]

Thirteen valent pneumococcal conjugate vaccine in Adults From 2008 through 2013, researchers conducted a randomized, placebo-controlled trial (community-acquired pneumonia immunization trial in adults [CAPiTA] trial) in the Netherlands among approximately 85,000 adults aged 65 years or older. It demonstrated

- 46% efficacy against vaccine-type pneumococcal pneumonia
- 45% efficacy against vaccine-type nonbacteremic pneumococcal pneumonia
- 75% efficacy against vaccine-type IPD[26]

PPSV23 More than 80% of healthy adults who receive PPSV23 develop antibodies against the serotypes contained in the vaccine. This immune response usually occurs within 2 to 3 weeks after vaccination. Older adults and persons with some chronic ill-nesses or immunodeficiency may not respond as well. Elevated antibody levels persist for at least 5 years in healthy adults but decline more quickly in persons with certain underlying illnesses. Children aged younger than 2 years generally have a poor anti-body response to PPSV23.[26]

Multiple studies have resulted in various estimates of the clinical effectiveness of PPSV23. Overall, the vaccine is 60% to 70% effective in preventing IPD caused by serotypes in the vaccine. PPSV23 shows reduced effectiveness among immuno-compromised persons; however, because of their increased risk of IPD, CDC rec-ommends PPSV23 for people who also receive PCV15 because of the broader serotype protection that PPSV23 provides. There is no consensus regarding the ability of PPSV23 to prevent nonbacteremic pneumococcal pneumonia. Studies comparing patterns of asymptomatic pneumococcal carriage before and after PPSV23 vaccination have not shown decreases in carriage rates among those vaccinated.[26]

Pneumococcal vaccine recommendations

CDC recommends pneumococcal vaccination for children aged younger than 5 years and adults aged 50 years or older.[27] CDC also recommends pneumococcal vaccina-tion for children and adults at an increased risk for pneumococcal disease. Follow the recommended immunization schedule to ensure that patients get the pneumococcal vaccines that they need. Immunization schedules change over time. Always refer to the CDC immunization schedules to ensure that the most current schedules are being followed. https://www.cdc.gov/vaccines/hcp/imz-schedules/index.html[27]

Catch-up guidance

Vaccinate children aged younger than 5 years who miss their shots or start the series later than recommended. The number of doses recommended and the intervals be-tween doses will depend on the child's age when vaccination begins.[27] The CDC has excellent job aids to assist in determining the appropriate number of doses based on the child's age and number of previous doses.[28] https://www.cdc.gov/vaccines/schedules/downloads/child/job-aids/pneumococcal.pdf[28]

Adults 50 years or older
- Administer PCV15, PCV20, or PCV21 for all adults 50 years or older
- Who have never received any PCV
- Whose previous vaccination history is unknown[29]

PCV15: additional vaccination needed for adults aged 65 years or older
- If PCV15 is used, administer a dose of PPSV23 1 year later. If PPSV23 is not available, 1 dose of PCV20 or PCV21 may be given. Only 1 dose of PPSV23 is

---

Box 4
Side effects of pneumococcal vaccines

- Feeling drowsy
- Loss of appetite
- Sore or swollen arm from the shot
- Fever
- Headache[33]

Table 1
Contraindications and precautions for pneumococcal vaccines

Vaccine	Contraindication	Precaution
PCV13, PCV15, and PCV20	Severe allergic reaction (eg, anaphylaxis) after a previous dose of PCV or any diphtheria-toxoid–containing vaccine or diphtheria-toxoid–containing vaccine or to a component of a vaccine (PCV or any diphtheria-toxoid–containing vaccine)[32]	Moderate or severe acute illness with or without fever
PPSV23	Severe allergic reaction (eg, anaphylaxis) after a previous dose or to a vaccine component	Moderate or severe acute illness with or without fever[32]

indicated. If previously administered, another dose is not needed. Once these conditions are met, pneumococcal vaccinations are complete.[29]

The minimum interval is 8 weeks and can be considered in adults with

- Immune compromising conditions
- Cochlear implant
- CSF leak

If the patient received PCV20 or PCV21, additional vaccination is not recommended. Shared clinical decision-making is recommended regarding the use of a supplemental PCV20 or PCV21 dose for adults aged 65 years or older who have completed their recommended vaccine series with both PCV13 and PPSV23. If PCV20 or PCV21 is used, a dose of PPSV23 is not indicated. Regardless of which vaccine is used (PCV20 or PCV21), their pneumococcal vaccinations are complete.[29]

The CDC has excellent job aids assist in determining the appropriate number of doses of pneumococcal vaccine for adults based on the age, condition and number, and type of doses previously received and shared clinical decision-making. CDC provides an excellent pneumococcal vaccine recommendations app for android and iPhone that can be downloaded: *PneumoRecs VaxAdvisor.*

Shared clinical decision-making:
https://www.cdc.gov/vaccines/hcp/admin/downloads/job-aid-SCDM-pneumococcal-508.pdf[30]

Pneumococcal Vaccine Timing for Adults:

Adult pneumococcal vaccine recommendations https://www.cdc.gov/pneumococcal/downloads/Vaccine-Timing-Adults-JobAid.pdf (**Box 4, Table 1**).[31]

SUMMARY

Pneumococcal infections cause a plethora of illness across the life span, but they particularly affect the very young and the very old. Pneumococcal vaccines have been available for years and updated formulations offer more opportunities to provide protection to individuals over a range of ages and conditions. Health care providers have the tools to provide these vaccines safely and effectively by following the CDC guidelines. While the schedules for these vaccines can appear confusing, CDC has developed effective tools to assist health care provider (HCPs) in determining the best practices for administration. Using this guidance, HCPs can offer protection to eligible individuals to offer effective protection against this dangerous and potentially life-threatening bacterium.

CLINICS CARE POINTS

- Always consult the CDC Immunizaton Schedules for most up to date recommendations for Pneumococcal vaccine for age and condition.
- Download CDC Vaccine Schedules app for iPhone or Android.
- Download PneumoRecs Vax Advisor app for iPhone or Android for assessment of adult pneumococcal vaccine indications.

DISCLOSURE

The author has no conflicts of interest to report.

REFERENCES

1. Gierke R, Wodi P, Kobayashi M. Pneumococcal disease. Centers for disease control and prevention. In: Hall E, Wodi AP, Hamborsky J, et al, editors. Epidemiology and prevention of vaccine-preventable diseases. 14th edition. Washington, DC: Public Health Foundation; 2021. Available at: https://www.cdc.gov/pinkbook/hcp/table-of-contents/chapter-17-pneumococcal-disease.html.
2. Runde TJ, Anjum F, Hafner JW. Bacterial meningitis. In: StatPearls [Internet]. Treasure Island (FL): StatPearls Publishing; 2024. Available at: https://www.ncbi.nlm.nih.gov/books/NBK470351/. Accessed August 8, 2023.
3. CDC. Pneumococcal disease. 2024. Available at: https://www.cdc.gov/pneumococcal/hcp/clinical-overview/index.html. Accessed September 21, 2024.
4. CDC. Invasive pneumococcal disease in young children before licensure of 13-valent pneumococcal conjugate vaccine — United States, 2007. MMWR Morb Mortal Wkly Rep 2010;59(9):253–7.
5. Richter SS, Heilmann KP, Dohrn CL, et al. Pneumococcal serotypes before and after introduction of conjugate vaccines, United States, 1999–2011. Emerg Infect Dis 2013;19(7):1074–83.
6. Pichichero M, Kaur R, Scott D, et al. Effectiveness of 13-valent pneumococcal conjugate vaccination for protection against acute otitis media caused by Streptococcus pneumoniae in healthy young children: a prospective observational study. Lancet Child Adolesc Health 2018;2(8):561–8.
7. Nowalk MP, Wateska AR, Lin CJ, et al. Racial disparities in adult pneumococcal vaccination indications and pneumococcal hospitalizations in the U.S. J Natl Med Assoc 2019;111(5):540–5.
8. Raman R, Brennan J, Ndi D, et al. Marked reduction of socioeconomic and racial disparities in invasive pneumococcal disease associated with conjugate pneumococcal vaccines. J Infect Dis 2021;223(7):1250–9.
9. CDC. Pneumococcal disease. Antibiotic-resistant Streptococcus pneumoniae. 2024. Available at: https://www.cdc.gov/pneumococcal/php/drug-resistance/index.html. Accessed September 28, 2024.
10. Dobay O. The complexity of serotype replacement of pneumococci. Hum Vaccines Immunother 2019;15(11):2725–8.
11. Tóthpál A, Desobry K, Joshi SS, et al. Variation of growth characteristics of pneumococcus with environmental conditions. BMC Microbiol 2019;19(1):304.
12. Kovács E, Sahin-Tóth J, Tóthpál A, et al. Vaccine-driven serotype-rearrangement is seen with latency in clinical isolates: comparison of carried and clinical

pneumococcal isolates from the same time period in Hungary. Vaccine 2019;37: 99–108.

13. Darrieux M, Goulart C, Briles D, et al. Current status and perspectives on protein-based pneumococcal vaccines. Crit Rev Microbiol 2015;41(2):190–200.

14. Lu YJ, Yadav P, Clements JD, et al. Options for inactivation, adjuvant, and route of topical administration of a killed, unencapsulated pneumococcal whole-cell vaccine. Clin Vaccine Immunol 2010;17:1005–12.

15. Rosch JW, Iverson AR, Humann J, et al. A live-attenuated pneumococcal vaccine elicits CD4+ T-cell dependent class switching and provides serotype independent protection against acute otitis media. EMBO Mol Med 2014;6:141–54.

16. McDaniel LS, Swiatlo E. Should pneumococcal vaccines eliminate nasopharyngeal colonization? mBio 2016;7(3). e00545-16.

17. Rappuoli R, De Gregorio E, Costantino P. On the mechanisms of conjugate vaccines. Proc Natl Acad Sci USA 2019;116(1):14–6.

18. Avery OT, Goebel WF. Chemo-immunological studies on conjugated carbohydrate-proteins: II. Immunological specificity of synthetic sugar-protein antigens. J Exp Med 1929;50:533–50.

19. Goebel WF, Avery OT. Chemo-immunological studies on conjugated carbohydrate-proteins: I. The synthesis of *p*-aminophenol beta-glucoside, *p*-aminophenol beta-galactoside, and their coupling with serum globulin. J Exp Med 1929;50: 521–31.

20. Costantino P, Viti S, Podda A, et al. Development and phase 1 clinical testing of a conjugate vaccine against meningococcus A and C. Vaccine 1992;10:691–8.

21. Obaro SK. The new pneumococcal vaccine. Clin Microbiol Infect 2002;8:623–33.

22. Moore MR, Link-Gelles R, Schaffner W, et al. Effect of use of 13-valent pneumococcal conjugate vaccine in children on invasive pneumococcal disease in children and adults in the USA: analysis of multisite, population-based surveillance. Lancet Infect Dis 2015;15(3):301–9.

23. Akkoyunlu M. State of pneumococcal vaccine immunity. Hum Vaccines Immunother 2024;20(1):2336358.

24. CDC. Pneumococcal disease surveillance and trends. 2024. Available at: https://www.cdc.gov/pneumococcal/php/surveillance/?CDC_AAref_Val=https://www.cdc.gov/pneumococcal/surveillance.html. Accessed September 28, 2024.

25. Berical AC, Harris D, Dela Cruz CS, et al. Pneumococcal vaccination strategies. An update and perspective. Ann Am Thorac Soc 2016;13(6):933–44.

26. CDC. About pneumococcal vaccines: for providers. 2024. Available at: https://www.cdc.gov/vaccines/vpd/pneumo/hcp/about-vaccine.html. Accessed September 30, 2024.

27. CDC. Vaccines and immunization schedules. 2024. Available at: https://www.cdc.gov/vaccines/hcp/imz-schedules/index.html. Accessed October 1, 2024.

28. CDC. Pneumococcal conjugate vaccine guidance. 2023. Available at: https://www.cdc.gov/vaccines/schedules/downloads/child/job-aids/pneumococcal.pdf. Accessed October 2, 2024.

29. CDC. Pneumococcal disease. Pneumococcal vaccine recommendations. 2024. Available at: https://www.cdc.gov/pneumococcal/hcp/vaccine-recommendations/index.html. Accessed October 3, 2024.

30. CDC. Shared clinical decision making. PCV20 or PCV21 vaccination for adults 65 Years or older. 2024. Available at: https://www.cdc.gov/vaccines/hcp/admin/downloads/job-aid-SCDM-pneumococcal-508.pdf. Accessed October 2, 2024.

31. CDC. Pneumococcal vaccine timing for adults. Available at: https://www.cdc. gov/pneumococcal/downloads/Vaccine-Timing-Adults-JobAid.pdf. Accessed October 3, 2024.

32. Advisory Committee on Immunization Practices. Preventing pneumococcal disease among infants and young children. Recommendations of the Advisory Committee on Immunization Practices (ACIP). MMWR Morb Mortal Wkly Rep 2000; 49(RR-9):1–3.

33. CDC. Pneumococcal vaccine safety. 2024. Available at: https://www.cdc.gov/ vaccine-safety/vaccines/pneumococcal.html?CDC_AAref_Val=https://www.cdc. gov/vaccinesafety/vaccines/pneumococcal-vaccine.html. Accessed September 30, 2024.

Respiratory Syncytial Virus in Focus
Emerging Research, Trends, and Clinical Implications

Clare Cardo McKegney, DNP, CPNP-PC[a,1],
Margaret Quinn, DNP, CPNP-PC, CPNP, CNE[b,*]

KEYWORDS

- Respiratory syncytial virus (RSV) • RSV prevention • RSV management

KEY POINTS

- RSV poses significant risks to infants aged under 6 months, especially those who are premature or have underlying health conditions.
- Recent advancements, including maternal vaccinations and monoclonal antibodies, offer promising strategies to reduce the global impact of RSV.
- The article focuses on the prevention of RSV, highlighting the latest breakthroughs aimed at protecting vulnerable populations.

INTRODUCTION

Respiratory syncytial virus (RSV) was first identified in 1956 and named because of the way in which the cells of the organism fuse to adjacent cells and create large multinucleated syncytia. This enveloped virus exists within the genus family of the Pneumovirus Paramyxoviridae. It is formed in a lipid layer surrounding a ribonucleoprotein core made up of several membrane proteins. It is a single-stranded RNA virus that consists of 11 proteins encoded by the 15.2 kb RSV genome.[1] The main function of such proteins is to attach to the host cells, which allows for replication.[2] As a nonsegmented genome, it is unlike influenza, and therefore, it does not have the capacity to mix and match its genetic code, which reduces the potential to cause large pandemics.[1] However, worldwide RSV continues to infect over 30 million children a year leading to bronchiolitis and pneumonia. In the United States, 50,000 to 80,000

Both authors contributed equally.
[a] Columbia University, School of Nursing, 560 West 168th Street, New York City, NY 10032, USA;
[b] Rutgers University, School of Nursing, 65 Bergen Street Rim 1138, Newark, NJ 07102, USA
[1] Present address: 16 Club Drive, Summit, NJ 07901.
* Corresponding author. 86 Raccoon Lane, Barnegat, NJ 08005.
E-mail address: Margaret.quinn@rutgers.edu

Nurs Clin N Am 60 (2025) 411–420
https://doi.org/10.1016/j.cnur.2024.10.002   nursing.theclinics.com
0029-6465/25/© 2024 Elsevier Inc. All rights reserved, including those for text and data mining, AI training, and similar technologies.

hospitalizations occur a year related to RSV.[3] Although there is only one serotype of RSV, there are 2 distinct strains "A" and "B." These strains are differentiated from the attachment proteins that exist within them, which is one of the contributing factors that can lead to the level of severity in disease.[2] While many children and adults who are infected with RSV fair well, the burden of the disease to children aged under 2 years and those with specific vulnerabilities can be severe. Therefore, the advances in prevention have become the focus of surrounding RSV.

BACKGROUND

The RSV virus is the leading cause of hospitalizations in infants aged less than 1 year in the United States. According to statistical findings in 2022, annually 33 million children worldwide were infected with RSV with over 100,000 deaths.[4] Assessment of such burden has been considered by number of hospitalizations, mortality and lower respiratory tract infections (LRTIs) that require medical attention. In the United States, RSV is predominantly seen in the winter to spring months with October being the start of RSV season throughout most of the country. In the years following the 2020 pandemic, the United States experienced a decrease in incidence initially, with a spike of the disease in the spring and summer months of 2021 to 2022.[5] It is reported that a more normal-appearing RSV season is expected for the 2024 to 2025 winter.[6] Morbidity and mortality are significantly higher in a subset of patients, including premature infants, patients with pre-existing cardiac, pulmonary, neurologic, and immunosuppressive disorders, and the elderly.[2] Until recently, much of the research dedicated to the RSV virus has been focused on treatment and management. With the current development of maternal vaccination and monoclonal antibodies (mAbs) for all infants, clinical practice providers are hopeful the stress of the virus may decrease over time.

CASE STUDY/PRESENTATION

A 2 month old child presents to the office with a runny nose, congestion, and cough for 2 days. Her mother reports today the infant has developed a fever of 101.3°F rectally and the cough has gotten worse, more frequent and sounds as if it is "choking her." The infant is breastfeeding every 3 hours, but overnight the feeding is more difficult. She is starting and stopping frequently to either cough or "catch her breath." Her mother reports she has had 6 wet diapers in 24 hours. She reports no change in her sleep although she is coughing while sleeping. Mother also reports that the 2 year old brother has a "cold." Upon examination, the provider finds the infant to be lying on the examination room table, alert with a loose staccato cough. She is febrile at the time of visit 101.4°F rectally. She appears in moderate amount of distress with respiratory rate of 66, heart rate of 112. Her examination reveals an alert infant, head, eyes, ears, nose, and throat examination reveals copious amount of thick mucoid clear nasal discharge, serous fluid noted to both tympanic membranes and watery eyes. Her lungs were appreciated to have diffuse expiratory wheeze. The infant was noted to be using accessory muscles for breathing with significant abdominal retractions. Her pulse oxygen was documented as 91% to 92% on room air. There was no rash reported. Point of service testing was positive for RSV.

The clinical presentation of this infant is a classic scenario that the pediatric provider encounters during the RSV season. Research suggests that by the age of 2 years most children have been infected with RSV and can and will be reinfected throughout their lifetime.[3] The virus causes similar symptoms of the common cold, making it hard to distinguish from another upper respiratory disease in the early stages. The clinical history of RSV in the early 2 to 5 days of illness is rhinorrhea and cough. Fever when present usually is low grade and typically noted in young infants and children who are naive to the virus. It is typically the cough that progresses to wheezing and difficulty breathing that brings families in for evaluation. Caregivers may also report poor infant feeding and in young children (aged 5 years and younger) with occasional vomiting and diarrhea.[7] When symptoms progress to lower airway involvement, the risk for apnea and cyanosis increases.

The physical examination of an infant with RSV infection can vary from mild to severe. Infants with congenital heart disease, history of prematurity, or underlying pulmonary disease may have more severe disease; children and adults with immunosuppression or chronic heart or lung disease and older adults, in general, are also at risk for severe disease.[7] Children with downs syndrome are at a higher risk of severe disease and complications.

RSV is known to invade the lower respiratory tract, thus being the most common pathogen to cause bronchiolitis. Bronchiolitis is a term that is used loosely; therefore, for the purpose of this article, it is important to recognize North American guidelines suggest that the diagnosis of bronchiolitis is reserved for children aged under 24 months who experience wheezing for the first time in the presence of an upper respiratory infection (URI).[8] The most common physical manifestations of acute RSV are rhinitis, cough, and coryza. A third of children infected will also have acute otitis media.[8] When the disease progresses to the lower respiratory tract, auscultation will reveal turbulent airflow with a prolonged expiratory wheeze, diffuse wheeze, and coarse breath sounds. Cough can worsen with retractions, feeding difficulties can develop, and tachypnea with the use of accessory muscles are often reported.[9] Infants aged less than 3 months are the most vulnerable to severe disease. Unfortunately, there are no accepted or validated tools to assist in the prediction of severe disease.[9] An accurate history and physical examination aid in the clinician's ability to recognize the disease's severity to develop the appropriate treatment plan.

The treatment of RSV bronchiolitis continues to be supportive. The 2014 American Academy of Pediatrics (AAP) clinical practice guidelines continue to be the most up to date management for clinicians in the primary care setting (**Table 1**). Within the practice setting, clinicians should encourage the patient to have adequate hydration at home and support the use of hypertonic saline nebulized solution as this may reduce hospitalization.[9] However, in the presence of inadequate feeding or fluid intake, apnea, lethargy, or moderate-to-severe respiratory distress (nasal flaring, tachypnea, grunting, retractions, or cyanosis), and/or a transcutaneous oxygen saturation of 92% or less in room air, hospitalization must be considered.

RSV bronchiolitis is a self-limiting disease that overall has a good prognosis. The majority of deaths observed is in infants aged less than 6 months and those with the risk factors stated earlier. Although symptoms usually resolve in 14 days, up to 40% of children with RSV bronchiolitis will have wheezing episodes through the first 5 years of their life.[10] Although there is not a cure, advances in preventative strategies have become the focus of RSV research.

RECOMMENDATIONS ON PREVENTION

There is currently no preventative option for RSV for all infants and can be based on primary and secondary prophylaxes.[10] Primary prophylaxis is based on handwashing and other hygienic measures such as disinfecting areas, limiting the risk of exposure, and using face masks with known symptoms.[11] Secondary prophylaxis can be from

Table 1
Common management of the RSV patient in the primary care setting

Considerations from the AAP Clinical Practice Guidelines	
Management Options	Rationale
Hydration	• Breastfeeding and bottle-feeding should be encouraged in small frequent feeds to ensure adequate hydration at home • Fluid replacement often is necessary when dehydration occurs secondary to difficulty breathing. Infants who are consuming <50% of their normal fluid intake may need nasogastric feeding
Antipyretics	• The use of antipyretic in the presence of fever of 100.4°F great for comfort is recommended
Saline nasal drops and nasal suctioning	• Simple nasal irrigation with frequent superficial suctioning can reduce the build of nasal mucus and improve work of breathing[8]
Oxygen therapy	• Apnea and decreased oxygenation are commonly seen in moderate-to-severe RSV bronchiolitis • Infants who maintain a Po_2 of <92% and increased work of breathing should be considered for supplemental oxygen • Preferred method of oxygen supplementation is via high flow nasal cannula and or continuous positive pressure[9]
Radiographs	• Chest radiographs are not routinely suggested in the diagnosis and management of RSV bronchiolitis
Bronchodilators, prolonged epinephrine, corticosteroids, and chest physiotherapy	• Most acute RSV bronchiolitis patients do not show any improvement in wheezing with the use of these therapies • These management options are noted to improve airway function in the asthmatic; however, they do not improve lung function or shorten the course of the illness when compared to hydration, inhaled saline solution, and supplemental oxygen when indicated
Antibiotics	• Antibiotics are not indicated in the treatment of RSV bronchiolitis • When comorbid infection such as an acute otitis media and or pneumonia are suspected then antibiotic therapy is warranted

Ralston et al (2014).[32]

mAbs and with other new developments including maternal vaccines to protect infants during the first months of life; single dose long-acting mAbs; and pediatric vaccination for widespread use (**Table 2**).

Maternal Vaccination

Maternal vaccination has proven successful for other childhood illnesses such as pertussis and influenza, which can provide protection from these pathogens.[12] Pertussis maternal vaccination programs have been well established, but the affliction of RSV through the first year of life, seasonality, and conditions of births from

Table 2
Summary of current secondary prophylaxis for respiratory syncytial virus for maternal child protection

	Immunization Approach	Generic Trade Name	Considerations
Maternal vaccination	Bivalent RSVpreF vaccine	RSV vaccine *Abrysvo*	• Single dose during 32–36 wk of pregnancy • September through January • Offers protection of the neonate from birth
mAbs	Short-acting mAb	Palivizumab *Synagis* (Sweeden)	• Infants born <29 wk and aged 12 mo old or younger at the beginning of RSV season • Comorbidities: cardiac and respiratory cardiovascular • 5 intramuscular doses • Increased cost
	Long-acting mAb	Nirsevimab-alip *Beyfortus* (Sweeden)	• Available to all newborns in their first RSV season • One intramuscular dose • Rapid and direct protection • Provides at least 5 mo of protection
Pediatric vaccines	Not universally available		• In clinical trials for older infants and children

Arexvy (respiratory syncytial virus vaccine adjuvanted) is not recommended for persons of childbearing age, and it is available for persons aged 60 y or older.

prematurity affect the timing of passage of maternal antibodies to the fetus for universal recommendations.[13] Additional differences have been noted in transplacental antibody transfer of RSV in both small for gestational age and large for gestational age infants.[14] Lastly, unlike influenza and pertussis, maternal protection from an RSV vaccine is unknown. RSV does not cause significant infection in otherwise healthy adults, so the overall benefit to pregnant persons is unknown.[15] Some reports state there is a greater risk of early cesarean delivery as well as adverse pregnancy outcomes in pregnant persons who are RSV positive, especially within the third trimester.[16]

There were several large clinical trials underway for maternal immunization. In a study funded by Novavax and the Bill and Melinda Gates Foundation (Clinical Trial MCT02624947), healthy pregnant women were randomized to receive a single dose of RSV fusion (F) protein nanoparticle vaccine or placebo between weeks 28 and 36 of pregnancy. A total of 4636 women underwent randomization, and there were 4579 live births.[17] During the first 90 days of life, there was a medically significant LRTI rate of 1.5% in the vaccine group and 2.4% in the placebo group. Hospitalizations for RSV-associated LRTI were 2.1% and 3.7%, respectively.[17] This study did not meet the prespecified success criterion for efficacy against RSV-associated, medically significant LRTI in infants up to 90 days of life, and further studies were encouraged.

An alternate phase III randomized double-blind study by GlaxoSmithKlein (Clinical Trial NCT04605159) was terminated early after the observation of higher risk of preterm birth in the vaccine group than the placebo group occurred.[18] The preliminary results suggested medically assessed RSV were lower in the dyads who received the maternal vaccine than placebo, but the risk of preterm birth was higher in the vaccine group.[18]

The American College of Obstetricians and Gynecologists published a Practice Advisory in late 2023 supporting Maternal Respiratory Syncytial Virus Vaccination.[19] This Practice Advisory provided guidance of the bivalent RSVpreF vaccine (trade name Abrysvo) by Pfizer (New York, NY). This is the only RSV vaccine approved by the United States Food and Drug Administration (FDA) and recommended by the Centers for Disease Control and Prevention (CDC). Pregnant people are suggested to receive a single dose during weeks 32 through 36 of pregnancy between September and January. It is disclosed in clinical trials there were more preterm births in the group that received Abrysvo although it is not confirmed if it is related to the vaccine.[20] Promising results stated Abrysvo decreased the risk of severe LRTI in infants by 81.8% within 90 days after birth and 69.4% within 180 days after birth.[20,21]

Monoclonal Antibodies

The mechanism of action of mAbs provides passive prophylaxis. Palivizumab, the novel mAbs, was licensed in 1998 by the FDA for high-risk infants for severe disease from RSV and provides a short half-life, which requires monthly injections.[22] The AAP published guidelines for the use of palivizumab, most recently updated in 2014, and the same guidelines are currently endorsed.[23] These guidelines indicate palivizumab for infants born 29 weeks' gestation or less and who are aged 12 months or younger at the beginning of RSV season with specific cardiac, respiratory, or neuromuscular comorbidities.[23] This mAb is injected in the outpatient setting during the RSV season for approximately 5 doses. Palivizumab does not prevent RSV, but can decrease hospitalizations, additional complications, and prevent LRTI. Palivizumab is quite costly requiring 5 doses through the RSV season with an estimated cost of US$11,320.[24]

The change in the AAP guidelines in 2014 recommended against the use of palivizumab in preterm infants born 29 0/7 weeks or later without additional risk factors due to cost-effectiveness concerns.[24] This caused a treatment gap in care for premature infants for RSV prophylaxis, with a subsequent rise in hospitalization rates and severity since this change.[25]

A new prophylaxis option is now available, which is both efficacious and cost-effective. Nirsevimab-alip (trade name Beyfortus by Sandolfi) provides direct and rapid protection lasting at least 5 months after administration.[15] A single administered injection before the RSV season protected healthy late preterm (>35 weeks) and term infants from RSV infections and RSV-associated LRTI the requirements of monthly injections.[26] Clinical trials noted a reduction of over 70% in patients given niservimab-alip compared to placebo.[27] There is a significant cost difference for the single injection at US$1748,[24] and nirsevimab-alip is noted to be 4 times more potent than palivizumab. Nirsevimab-alip is available as part of the Vaccine for Children program as well as private insurance with limited restrictions.[28] A shortage of the mAb was noted in 2023 resulting in an increase in RSV hospitalizations, and the CDC expedited delivery of additional doses to be distributed.[27] No current data are available for the 2024 season at the time of publication.

Pediatric Vaccines for Older Infants and Children

There is no licensed RSV vaccine for pediatric patients. A prototype of a formalin-inactivated RSV vaccine was tested in the 1960s, but testing was stopped due to the lack of efficacy and noted disease-enhanced symptoms following exposure to RSV leading to the death of several participants.[29] There are numerous variations of different antigens and vaccine formats being tested, and they vary by target group (newborns, children, pregnant women, and the elderly).[29] In 2023, the FDA approved the first RSV vaccine for individuals aged 60 years and older. Arexvy (GSK - GlaxoSmithKlein, Belgium), a lyophilized recombinant RSV glycoprotein F, stimulates the production of neutralizing antibodies by activating humoral and cellular immune responses and forms memory B and T cells, and it is not approved for those aged less than 50 years.[30]

Infants infected with a natural RSV infection have not shown to have a strong immune response less than 18 months of age,[31] which poses significant challenges within infant vaccine development for RSV related to the inability for infants to generate long-term immune responses following immunization or infection due to the need for a mature immune system to develop an immune response.[15] Infants born during the RSV season are especially vulnerable, and current testing of the vaccinations may help children through their second RSV season. Several vaccines are being researched, but none are targeting newborns.[15,31]

Vaccines for Older Adults

Preventive vaccination is recommended for older adults at risk for complications from RSV. Older persons with chronic heart or lung disease, those who are immunocompromised, persons in long-term care, and persons with other chronic diseases should be vaccinated. Clinicians should refer to the CDC guidelines for the most up-to-date recommendations for RSV vaccinations in older adults.

SUMMARY

RSV remains a significant public health concern, especially for infants, young children, and the elderly. Globally, RSV is the leading cause of hospitalization, with over 33 million diagnoses and approximately 100,000 deaths annually. Despite these alarming statistics, there is no universal prevention plan in place. The presentation of RSV ranges from mild URIs to severe respiratory distress, affecting both premature and full-term infants alike. Healthy newborns are particularly at risk, with up to 75% of RSV-related hospitalizations and one-quarter of associated deaths occurring in this group.

However, new preventative measures for the 2024 RSV season offer hope. These advancements include updated maternal vaccines, mAbs like nirsevimab-alip, and improved diagnostic tools aimed at early detection and enhanced immunity. While vaccines for infants and young children are not yet commercially available, an approved vaccine for pregnant women is now in use, promoting transplacental antibody transfer to protect newborns. Ongoing research is needed to fully understand the efficacy, duration, and impact of this approach on newborns. Although high-risk infants (around 7% of all newborns) benefit from short-acting mAbs,[15] the broader application of long-acting mAbs could significantly reduce the RSV burden for the healthy newborn population as well. With these new interventions, including public health strategies aimed at reducing transmission and hospitalization rates, the outlook on RSV prevention is promising. As we move forward, the public health community anticipates a substantial reduction in RSV-related illness, particularly in vulnerable infant populations, marking a critical step in the global effort to control respiratory diseases.

DISCLOSURE

The authors declare no conflicts of interest related to the content of this article. There is no financial support or affiliations related to the content of this article.

REFERENCES

1. Jha A, Jarvis H, Fraser C, et al. Respiratory syncytial virus. In: Hui DS, Rossi GA, Johnston SL, editors. SARS, MERS and other viral lung infections. Chapter 5. European Respiratory Society; 2016. Available at: https://www.ncbi.nlm.nih.gov/books/NBK442240/.
2. Jain H, Schweitzer JW, Justice NA. Respiratory syncytial virus infection in children. In: StatPearls. Treasure Island (FL): StatPearls Publishing; 2024. Available at: https://www.ncbi.nlm.nih.gov/books/NBK459215/.
3. Cieslak C. Nirsevimab immunization to prevent respiratory syncytial virus–associated lower respiratory tract infections in infants and children up to 24 months of age. Nursing for Womens Health 2024;28(1):75–9.
4. Binns E, Tuckerman J, Licciardi P, et al. Respiratory syncytial virus, recurrent wheeze, and asthma: a narrative review of pathophysiology, prevention, and future directions. J Paediatr Child Health 2022;58(10):16197.
5. Chuang YC, Lin KP, Wang LA, et al. The impact of the COVID-19 pandemic on respiratory syncytial virus infection: a narrative review. Infect Drug Resist 2023;16:661–75.
6. Centers for Disease Control and Prevention (CDC). 2024-2025 respiratory disease season outlook. 2024. Available at: https://www.cdc.gov/cfa-qualitative-assessments/php/data-research/season-outlook24-25/index.html.
7. Colosia A, Costello J, McQuarrie K, et al. Systematic literature review of the signs and symptoms of respiratory syncytial virus. Influenza Other Respir Viruses 2023;17(2). https://doi.org/10.1111/irv.13100.
8. Ghazaly M, Nadel S. Overview of prevention and management of acute bronchiolitis due to respiratory syncytial virus. Expert Rev Anti Infect Ther 2018;16(12):913–28.

9. Oppenlander KE, Chung AA, Clabaugh D. Respiratory syncytial virus bronchiolitis: rapid evidence review. Am Fam Physician 2023;108(1):52–7.

10. Jartti T, Smits HH, Bønnelykke K, et al. Bronchiolitis needs a revisit: distinguishing between virus entities and their treatments. Allergy 2019;74(1):40–52.

11. Centers for Disease Control and Prevention (CDC). About RSV. 2024. Available at: https://www.cdc.gov/rsv/about/index.html.

12. Gkentzi D, Katsakiori P, Marangos M, et al. Maternal vaccination against pertussis: a systematic review of the recent literature. Arch Dis Child Fetal Neonatal Ed 2017;102(5). https://doi.org/10.1136/archdischild-2016-312341.

13. Engmann C, Fleming JA, Khan S, et al. Closer and closer? maternal immunization: current promise, future horizons. J Perinatol 2020;40(6):844–57.

14. Yildiz M, Kara M, Sutcu M, et al. Evaluation of respiratory syncytial virus IgG antibody dynamics in mother-infant pairs cohort. Eur J Clin Microbiol Infect Dis 2020; 39(7):1279–86.

15. Baraldi E, Checcucci Lisi G, Costantino C, et al. RSV disease in infants and young children: can we see a brighter future? Hum Vaccines Immunother 2022; 18(4):2079322.

16. Hause AM, Panagiotakopoulos L, Weintraub ES, et al. Adverse outcomes in pregnant women hospitalized with respiratory syncytial virus infection: a case series. Clin Infect Dis 2021;72(1):138–40.

17. Madhi SA, Polack FP, Piedra PA, et al. Respiratory syncytial virus vaccination during pregnancy and effects in infants. N Engl J Med 2020;383(5):426–39.

18. Dieussaert I, Hyung Kim J, Luik S, et al. RSV prefusion F protein-based maternal vaccine: preterm birth and other outcomes. N Engl J Med 2024;390(11):1009–21.

19. American College of Obstetricians and Gynecologists (ACOG). Maternal respiratory syncytial virus infection: prevention and management guidelines. ACOG Practice Advisory 2024. Available at: https://www.acog.org.

20. Kampmann B, Madhi SA, Munjal I, et al. Respiratory syncytial virus vaccine during pregnancy and effects in infants. N Engl J Med 2023;388(16):1451–64.

21. Fleming-Dutra KE, Jones JM, Roper LE, et al. Use of the Pfizer respiratory syncytial virus vaccine during pregnancy for the prevention of respiratory syncytial virus-associated lower respiratory tract disease in infants: recommendations of the Advisory Committee on Immunization Practices - United States, 2023. MMWR Morb Mortal Wkly Rep 2023;72(41):1115–22.

22. Clark RH, Tolia VN, Ahmad KA. Palivizumab use in the NICU: 1999–2020. Pediatrics 2022;150(1). https://doi.org/10.1542/peds.2021-055607.

23. Caserta MT, O'Leary ST, Munoz FM, et al. Palivizumab prophylaxis in infants and young children at increased risk of hospitalization for respiratory syncytial virus infection. Pediatrics 2023;152(1). https://doi.org/10.1542/peds.2023-061803.

24. Yu T, Padula WV, Yieh L, et al. Cost-effectiveness of nirsevimab and palivizumab for respiratory syncytial virus prophylaxis in preterm infants. Pediatrics 2024; 153(1). https://doi.org/10.1542/peds.2023-061805.

25. Krilov LR, Fergie J, Goldstein M. Impact of the 2014 American Academy of Pediatrics immunoprophylaxis policy on the rate, severity, and cost of respiratory syncytial virus hospitalizations among preterm infants. Am J Perinatol 2020;37(2): 174–83.

26. Griffin MP, Yuan Y, Takas T, et al. Single-dose nirsevimab for prevention of RSV in preterm infants. N Engl J Med 2020;383(5):415–25.

27. Rahmat ZS, Ahmad S, Malikzai A. CDC changes recommendations due to severe nirsevimab shortage during the 2023-2024 RSV season. Pediatr Pulmonol 2024; 59(4):1108–9.

28. Sanofi. How to get Beyfortus at no cost to you. 2024. Available at: https://www.beyfortus.com/about/cost-and-coverage.

29. Biagi C, Dondi A, Scarpini S, et al. Current state and challenges in developing respiratory syncytial virus vaccines. Vaccines (Basel) 2020;8(4):672.

30. Awosika AO, Patel P. Respiratory syncytial virus prefusion F (RSVPreF3) vaccine. In: StatPearls. Treasure Island (FL): StatPearls Publishing; 2024. Available at: https://www.ncbi.nlm.nih.gov/books/NBK594261/.

31. Esposito S, Scarselli E, Lelii M, et al. Antibody response to respiratory syncytial virus infection in children <18 months old. Hum Vaccines Immunother 2016; 12(7):1700–6.

32. Ralston SL, Lieberthal AS, Meissner HC, et al. Clinical practice guideline: the diagnosis, management, and prevention of bronchiolitis. Pediatrics 2014;134(5): e1474–502.

Measles Matters
A Clinical Overview and Update

Angela Otto-Ryan, DNP, CPNP-PC, CBC[a],*,
Jeffrey Kwong, DNP, MPH, AGPCNP-BC[b,c]

KEYWORDS

- Measles • Rubeola • Vaccine-preventable diseases • Epidemiology • Immunization
- Infectious disease

KEY POINTS

- Highly infectious yet preventable: Measles is a highly transmissible viral infection that may result in life-threatening complications, yet it is preventable through routine vaccination.
- Epidemiology and transmission: Transmission occurs through respiratory droplets and airborne particles and a 95% immunization rate is required to maintain herd immunity within a population.
- Clinical presentation and complications: Clinical manifestations include fever, cough, and a characteristic maculopapular rash, with potential complications such as pneumonia, encephalitis, acute disseminated encephalomyelitis, and subacute sclerosing panencephalitis.
- Laboratory Testing and Management: Diagnosis is confirmed through reverse transcription-polymerase chain reaction and serologic testing, with therapeutic interventions focused on supportive care and vitamin A supplementation.
- Prevention and Immunization: The most effective strategy for measles prevention is immunization, with 2 appropriately timed doses of the measles, mumps, and rubella vaccine shown to confer long-lasting, comprehensive protection.

INTRODUCTION

Measles is an extremely contagious viral illness, caused by a paramyxovirus of the genus *Morbillivirus*.[1] It is a serious and highly transmissible illness that can be life-threatening, but is preventable through vaccination. Prior to the development of measles vaccine in the 1960s, the disease was one of the primary causes of illness and death among children worldwide.[2] As one of the world's most virulent diseases, measles has an estimated basic reproduction number between 12 and 18, meaning

[a] Division of Entry to Baccalaureate Practice, Rutgers University School of Nursing, Newark, NJ, USA; [b] Division of Advanced Nursing Practice, Rutgers University School of Nursing, 65 Bergen Street, Suite 1132A, Newark, NJ 07107, USA; [c] NYU Langone Health, 360 W 31st Street, 3rd Floor, New York, NY 10001, USA
* Corresponding author. 180 University Avenue, Office 262, Newark, NJ 07102.
E-mail address: amo126@sn.rutgers.edu

Nurs Clin N Am 60 (2025) 421–429
https://doi.org/10.1016/j.cnur.2025.04.001
0029-6465/25/© 2025 Elsevier Inc. All rights reserved, including those for text and data mining, AI training, and similar technologies.

Abbreviations	
ADEM	Acute disseminated encephalomyelitis
AIIR	airborne infection isolation room
CDC	Centers for Disease Control and Prevention
MMR	measles, mumps, and rubella
MMRV	measles, mumps, rubella, and varicella
RT-PCR	reverse-transcription polymerase chain reaction

1 infected individual can spread the virus to 12 to 18 others in a population with no prior immunity, making it more contagious than influenza or pertussis.[3] Beyond its highly contagious nature, the measles virus can weaken the host's immune system, making individuals more vulnerable to secondary infections, predominantly those affecting the respiratory and gastrointestinal systems.[4] Despite global vaccination efforts, measles continues to be widespread and deadly in many low-resource countries. According to the World Health Organization, approximately 142,300 measles-related deaths occurred worldwide in 2018.[1] In the United States, several outbreaks have also been reported in recent years. The current measles outbreak, as of April 3, 2025, has resulted in 607 confirmed measles cases reported across 22 US jurisdictions, including Alaska, California, Colorado, Florida, Georgia, Kansas, Kentucky, Maryland, Michigan, Minnesota, New Jersey, New Mexico, New York City, New York State, Ohio, Oklahoma, Pennsylvania, Rhode Island, Tennessee, Texas, Vermont, and Washington.[5]

Epidemiology

Measles is an exclusively human infection, with no identified animal reservoir. The virus relies solely on humans for transmission.[1] Measles spreads from person-to-person via large respiratory droplets and secretions, as well as through aerosolized airborne particles that can remain in enclosed spaces, for up to 2 hours after an infected person has left.[1] The incubation period typically ranges from 10 to 14 days, but may extend up to 23 days in some cases.[6] Symptoms can last up to 3 weeks, and individuals are considered contagious from approximately 4 days before the rash appears to about 4 days afterward.[1,6] Due to measles' highly infectious nature, achieving and sustaining herd immunity requires at least 95% of the population to receive 2 doses of a measles-containing vaccine.[6]

Measles has historically been considered a childhood illness, and prior to the introduction of widespread vaccination, was responsible for over 4 million deaths annually across the globe.[6] In areas where immunization rates remain low, children continue to be the most impacted group, often resulting in significant mortality.[6] The case-fatality rate can vary based on several factors, including vaccination rates within the population, the age at which individuals contract the infection, overall nutritional status, the prevalence of HIV, and the overall effectiveness of a health care system.[6] As these conditions evolve, the case-fatality ratio may also shift over time.

Pathophysiology

The genome of the measles virus is composed of single-stranded, negative-sense RNA and shares a close genetic relationship with the viruses responsible for rinderpest and canine distemper.[1] Two envelope proteins play key roles in the virus's ability to cause disease: the fusion (F) protein facilitates the merging of viral and host cell membranes, enabling viral entry and contributing to cell damage, while the hemagglutinin (H) protein allows the virus to attach to specific receptors on host cells.[1] The measles virus initiates infection by attaching to 2 specific receptors: CD150 (also known as

SLAM) and nectin-4.[6] CD150 is primarily expressed on various immune cells, including immature thymocytes, memory and activated T cells, naive and activated B cells, macrophages, and dendritic cells.[6] Nectin-4, on the other hand, is located on the basal surface of epithelial cells within the respiratory tract, particularly at adherens junctions.[6]

Once the measles virus enters the respiratory tract, it is taken up by macrophages and dendritic cells, which then pass the virus to immune cells such as thymocytes, T and B lymphocytes, and hematopoietic stem cells (**Fig. 1**).[6] These infected mononuclear cells serve as vehicles for transporting the virus to various nonlymphoid tissues, where it replicates within epithelial and endothelial cells. This phase of widespread viral dissemination occurs without noticeable symptoms and typically spans 7 to 14 days.[6] In the early, prodromal stage of measles, individuals typically develop a fever along with at least one of the following symptoms: cough, runny nose, or eye inflammation.[6] These symptoms result from damage to epithelial cells caused by viral replication. The hallmark rash of measles, a maculopapular eruption, appears as part of the body's immune response to the virus and is observed in nearly all individuals with a healthy immune system.[6] Keratinocyte infection relies on the presence of nectin-4 and may lead to keratoconjunctivitis, which in severe cases can cause blindness.[6] As immune cells infiltrate and begin eliminating the measles-infected lymphoid and myeloid cells, the resulting immune reaction leads to the development of the characteristic rash, along with hyperemia and tissue swelling.[6]

During the acute phase of measles infection, individuals experience significant, though typically temporary, immune suppression, increasing their vulnerability to additional infections. While the virus triggers robust humoral and cellular immune responses that generally lead to lifelong immunity against measles itself, research indicates it may also disrupt the normal balance of lymphocyte populations.[6] This phenomenon, known as immune amnesia, results in a considerable loss of preexisting immune memory.[6] The decline in antibody-based immunity can persist for months or even years, leaving affected individuals more susceptible to other infectious diseases

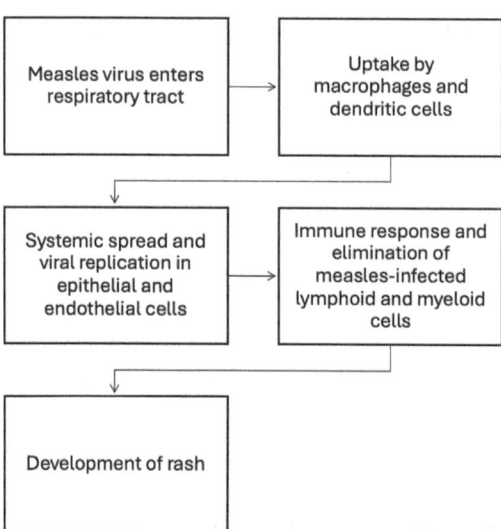

Fig. 1. Pathophysiology of measles. (*From* Sonia L, Sharma S. Medical-surgical nursing prep manual for undergraduates volume-I. Elsevier, 2016. Figure 95.1.)

over an extended period. Immunization against measles helps preserve existing immune memory that might otherwise be diminished by natural measles infection; it also protects against potential complications arising from subsequent infections by other pathogens.[6]

Clinical Presentation

The incubation period for measles, from the time of exposure to the onset of early symptoms, typically spans 11 to 12 days.[1] On average, the rash appears about 14 days after initial exposure, although the timeline can range from 7 to 21 days.[1] The initial prodromal phase of illness generally lasts between 2 to 4 days, but can extend from 1 to 7 days.[1] This stage is marked by a progressively rising fever, often reaching temperatures between 103°F and 105°F, along with a combination of cough, nasal congestion, and coryza.[1]

A distinctive feature of early measles is the appearance of Koplik spots (**Fig. 2**), which are tiny blue-white lesions on a bright red background, typically found inside the cheek (buccal mucosa).[1] These spots emerge 1 to 2 days before the rash and are considered a unique, although not always reliable, indicator of measles.

The measles rash (**Fig. 3**) is characterized by flat and slightly raised red lesions (maculopapular) and usually persists for 5 to 6 days.[1] It begins at the hairline and then spreads to the face and neck before gradually progressing downward to the trunk, arms, legs, and eventually the hands and feet. The rash usually spreads over a period of 3 days.[1] Early in the course of the rash, the lesions may temporarily fade when pressed (blanching), but by days 3 to 4, this blanching typically disappears.[1] In more affected areas, the rash may later peel as it resolves. The fading of the exanthem follows the same cephalocaudal sequence, begining from the head and ending at the extremities. Other common symptoms include loss of appetite and widespread swelling of lymph nodes.[1]

Traditionally, measles is clinically suspected in patients who present with fever, a spreading maculopapular rash, and at least one of the following: cough, conjunctivitis, or coryza.[6] However, individuals who have been vaccinated may exhibit a much milder form of the disease, or no symptoms at all, a condition referred to as modified measles.[6] This variation in presentation suggests that in highly immunized populations, a more flexible clinical case definition may be necessary to ensure proper detection of cases. Additionally, individuals with weakened immune systems may fail to develop hallmark signs such as rash or conjunctivitis, making diagnosis more

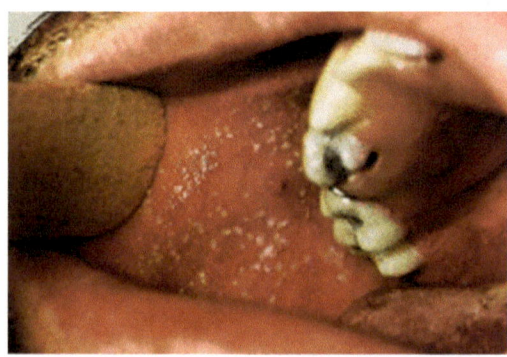

Fig. 2. Koplik's spots. (*From* Emond RT, Welsby PD, Rowland HA, editors. Color atlas of infectious diseases. 4th edition. Mosby; 2003.)

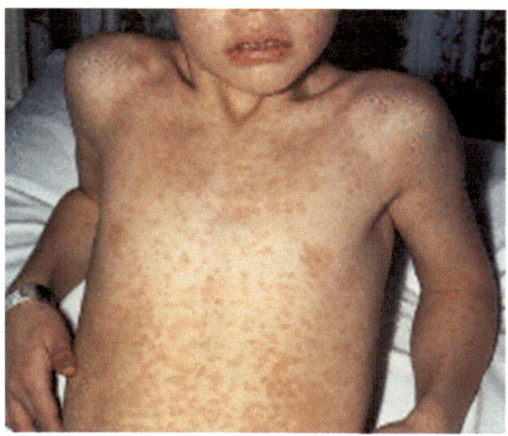

Fig. 3. Measles rash. (*From* Hobson RP. Infectious disease. In: Walker BR, Colledge NR, Ralston SH, et al, editors. Davidson's principles and practice of medicine. 22nd edition. Elsevier; 2014.)

difficult. Although Koplik spots have long been regarded as a defining clinical feature of measles, recent evaluations have questioned their reliability as a consistent diagnostic marker.[6] Relying solely on clinical symptoms is not sufficient for an accurate diagnosis, making laboratory testing essential for all suspected cases; this helps confirm the presence of measles, distinguish it from other illnesses, and reduce the risk of continued spread.

Laboratory Testing

Confirmation of measles infection can be done through laboratory testing. The Centers for Disease Control and Prevention (CDC) recommends performing reverse-transcription polymerase chain reaction (RT-PCR) testing of nasopharyngeal, throat, or urine specimens with concurrent serology testing for measles antibodies.[7] Some local public health jurisdictions may have different testing requirements, so clinicians should consult their local practice authority for guidance on diagnostic testing.

The timing and type of test used are important in confirming a measles diagnosis. RT-PCR tests are best done within 3 days of the appearance of rash because the level of viral RNA can decline after the rash appears. Although RT-PCR is best done early after the appearance of a rash, measles RNA may remain detectable on RT-PCR tests up to 10 days after rash onset.[8] Serology testing for antimeasles IgM antibodies typically becomes detectable by day 3 of the rash and can remain detectable for 6 to 8 weeks after acute measles. Serology specimens obtained less than 3 days after the presence of the rash may be negative. Therefore, clinicians may consider repeat testing if the initial sample was obtained early after rash appearance. Antimeasles IgG becomes detectable approximately 2 weeks after the appearance of the rash and remains positive indefinitely.

Clinical Management

There is no cure for measles, therefore, treatment is primarily supportive care. Given that patients experience fever and are prone to dehydration, care should focus on ensuring that patients maintain adequate hydration and receive antipyretics as needed. A recent analysis found that approximately 25% of persons hospitalized for measles were admitted due to dehydration.[9]

Additionally, the American Academy of Pediatrics recommends that persons with measles receive 2 doses of vitamin A, regardless of hospitalization status, to prevent complications (**Table 1**).[10] Vitamin A deficiency can lower immune function and is associated with greater morbidity and mortality in persons with measles. Vitamin A is not intended for measles prevention and should not be administered in high doses, as this can result in toxicity. Symptoms of vitamin A toxicity may include nausea, vomiting, headaches, fatigue, joint and bone pain, blurred vision, skin and hair changes, increased intracranial pressure, liver damage, confusion, and even coma.[10]

Complications

Complications associated with measles infection can impact a variety of body systems. Patients may experience diarrhea, otitis media, pneumonia, keratitis, myocarditis, and neurologic complications. Many of the more common respiratory or gastrointestinal complications are due to secondary bacterial infection caused by pathogens such as S. *pneumoniae*, H. *influenzae* type B, or staphylococci.[11] Secondary viral infections have been documented and include parainfluenza, adenovirus, respiratory syncytial virus, cytomegalovirus, enterovirus, and influenza.[11] There is data on the use of ribavirin in measles pneumonia; however, its use remains controversial. Clinicians are encouraged to consult with an infectious disease expert if considering ribavirin in persons with measles-related pneumonia.[8]

Several neurologic complications can occur with measles. Encephalitis has been estimated to occur in approximately 1 per 1000 cases and can be seen within 5 days of rash onset (range 1–14 days). However, it is important to note that there have been cases of encephalitis occurring in persons without the typical measles rash.[11] Patients with encephalitis may experience fever, seizure, vomiting, stiff neck, meningeal irritation, coma, or other neurologic deficits. Acute disseminated encephalomyelitis (ADEM), another neurologic complication, is characterized by classic encephalitis symptoms of fever, headache, seizures, but may also include altered mental status, coma, and motor dysfunction including paraplegia, or loss of bowel and bladder continence.[8] ADEM is seen in the recovery phase of measles within 2 weeks of the rash. Unfortunately, mortality due to ADEM is estimated to be 10% to 20%.

Subacute sclerosing panencephalitis is a rare long-term neurologic complication. Unlike other complications, this condition manifests an average of 7 years after initial measles infection.[8] Clinical symptoms include mild mental deterioration that progresses to seizures, motor disability, and a persistent vegetative state that ultimately leads to death within 1 to 3 years following diagnosis. This condition typically occurs in persons who acquire measles under the age of 2.

Table 1
Vitamin A dosing for persons with measles

Age	Dose
12 months or older	• 200 000 IU (60 000 µg retinol activity equivalent [RAE])
6 months - 11 months of age	• 100 000 IU (30 000 µg RAE)
Younger than 6 months of age	• 50 000 IU (15 000 µg RAE)
An additional (ie, a third) age-specific dose of vitamin A should be given 2 through 6 weeks later to children with clinical signs and symptoms of vitamin A deficiency	

Prevention

Immunization

Vaccination against measles is the best means of preventing the disease. There are 3 available vaccines licensed and approved in the United States that provide protection against measles. Two formulations of the vaccines offer protection against measles, mumps, and rubella (MMR) (the M-M-R-II vaccine developed by Merck & Co, Inc and Priorix developed by GlaxoSmithKline Biologicals).[12] Both of these products are interchangeable. A third vaccine, ProQuad, is a combination vaccine that provides protection against measles, mumps, rubella, and varicella (MMRV). The MMRV vaccine is not interchangeable with either of the 2 MMR vaccines. All vaccines are live-attenuated formulations.

The Advisory Committee on Immunization Practices (ACIP) recommends 2 doses of the MMR vaccine, with the initial dose given between the ages of 12 to 15 months, followed by a second dose given between the ages of 4 to 6 years of age.[13] Catch-up immunizations may be administered to individuals outside of the recommended immunization schedule. In these instances, or for adults in need of immunization, 2 doses of vaccine may be administered at least 4 weeks apart.[13] The MMRV vaccine can be used as an alternative, but the MMRV vaccine is approved only for children between the ages of 12 months through 12 years of age.

Adults born before 1957 are commonly presumed to be immune to measles due to likely exposure to natural infection.[13] Individuals vaccinated between 1963 and 1967 may have received an inactivated version of the measles vaccine, which has been found to be less effective than live-attenuated formulations. In these instances, persons may not have protective immunity. Adults who are not immune should receive 1 or 2 doses of MMR separated at least 4 weeks apart based on their medical history, unless there is a contraindication (eg, advanced immune suppression, severe allergy, or pregnancy). Serologic testing for measles IgG can be used to verify immunity.

The MMR and MMRV vaccines have been proven to be safe and effective. A single dose of MMR is 93% effective in reducing measles, and 2 doses of MMR is 97% effective in reducing infection.[13] There is no association between the MMR vaccine and autism.[12,13] The most common side effect of the vaccine is pain and tenderness at the injection site, fever, mild rash, and joint stiffness. Although immunization against measles is part of routine childhood preventive care, recent data from the CDC indicate that rates of vaccination among kindergartners decreased in the 2023 to 2024 school year to 92.7% of children vaccinated from 95.2% just 3 years earlier.[5] One of the vital roles nurses and nurse practitioners can play is in providing appropriate education to patients and parents of young children on the importance of vaccination. The CDC offers a variety of resources that health care providers can use to help educate patients and their families on vaccines available at https://www.cdc.gov/vaccines/hcp/resources/index.html.

Postexposure prophylaxis

For individuals without immunity to measles or who are severely immunocompromised, postexposure prophylaxis (PEP) should be offered if these individuals are exposed to measles. Two options for measles PEP are recommended. Immunoglobulin (dosed at 0.5 mg/kg, maximum dose of 15 mg), can be administered up to 6 days following exposure.[13] For nonimmune individuals without contraindication to the MMR vaccine, the vaccine should be given. Additionally, home quarantine is recommended for persons receiving immunoglobulin. Individuals should be advised to quarantine at home for 21 to 28 days, based on local health department guidelines.[14] The longer 28-day quarantine period is suggested for persons receiving immunoglobulin because the incubation period may be delayed in these individuals.

HEALTH CARE FACILITY PATIENT MANAGEMENT AND PREVENTION OF DISEASE

For patients with presumed or diagnosed measles seen within a health care facility (such as an outpatient office, emergency department, or inpatient unit), airborne precautions should be used.[15] Patients (and any accompanying caregivers) should be isolated from others and face masks should be placed on the patient and their caregivers. Ideally, patients should be placed in an airborne infection isolation room (AIIR).[15] If and AIIR not available, place the patient and accompanying caregivers in a single room with the door closed. If the patient must be transported outside of the isolation room, the patient should wear a mask. Airborne precautions may be discontinued 4 days after the presence of rash (with Day 0 being the first appearance of rash).[14] Airborne precautions may be extended for immunocompromised patients due to the risk of prolonged viral shedding. Care of the patient should be limited to health care personnel with evidence of immunity to measles. Health care personnel should adhere to their facility's policies regarding airborne precautions and decontamination after the patient is discharged.

SUMMARY

Measles is one of the most highly contagious, vaccine-preventable illnesses that has seen a growing resurgence in recent years. Although the infection is self-limiting, measles is associated with various complications, may lead to some long-term sequelae, and can result in mortality. Early recognition and infection control measures can limit the spread of the infection among those who remain vulnerable to the disease. Educating and ensuring all eligible individuals receive appropriate vaccination is critical in controlling and preventing the spread of this infection. Nurses play a key role in managing and preventing measles.

CLINICS CARE POINTS

- Prompt Recognition is Crucial: Early identification of prodromal symptoms (fever, cough, conjunctivitis, Koplik spots) enables timely isolation to reduce the risk of transmission, especially in clinical settings.
- Supportive Management Remains the Mainstay: There is no antiviral treatment. Measles care focuses on symptom relief, hydration, and nutritional support, with vitamin A recommended to reduce morbidity, particularly in young children.
- Monitor for Complications: Be vigilant for secondary bacterial infections, pneumonia, and neurologic sequelae, which may require hospitalization and multidisciplinary care.
- Vaccination History Matters: Always assess vaccination status during febrile rash illness evaluation. Underimmunization may increase individual risk and community vulnerability.

REFERENCES

1. Centers for Disease Control and Prevention (CDC). In: Hall E, Wodi AP, Hamborsky J, et al, editors. Epidemiology and prevention of vaccine-preventable diseases. 14th edition. Washington, DC: Public Health Foundation; 2021. Available

at: https://www.merle-arbeitsmedizin.de/wp-content/uploads/2022/02/CDC-Pink-Book-Version-14th-Edition.pdf. Accessed March 24, 2025.

2. Moss WJ. Measles. Lancet 2017;390(10111):2490–502.

3. Gastañaduy PA, Goodson JL, Panagiotakopoulos L, et al. Measles in the 21st century: progress toward achieving and sustaining elimination. J Infect Dis 2021;224(Suppl 4):S420–8.

4. Xia S, Gullickson CC, Metcalf CJE, et al. Assessing the effects of measles virus infections on childhood infectious disease mortality in Brazil. J Infect Dis 2022; 227(1):133–40.

5. Centers for Disease Control and Prevention (CDC). Measles cases and outbreaks. Available at: https://www.cdc.gov/measles/data-research/index.html. Accessed April 9, 2025.

6. Hübschen JM, Gouandjika-Vasilache I, Dina J. Measles. Lancet 2022;399-(10325):678–90.

7. Centers for Disease Control and Prevention (CDC). Clinical overview of measles. 2024. Available at: https://www.cdc.gov/measles/hcp/clinical-overview/. Accessed April 6, 2025.

8. Gans H, Maldanado YA. Measles: clinical manifestations, diagnosis, treatment, and prevention. 2025. Available at: https://www-uptodate-com.proxy.libraries. rutgers.edu/contents/measles-clinical-manifestations-diagnosis-treatment-and-prevention?search=measles%20&source=search_result&selectedTitle=1%7E150& usage_type=default&display_rank=1. Accessed April 6, 2025.

9. Chovatiya R, Silverberg JI. Inpatient morbidity and mortality of measles in the United States. PLoS One 2020;15(4):e0231329.

10. American Academy of Pediatrics. Measles frequently asked questions: does vitamin A prevent measles. 2025. Available at: https://www.aap.org/en/patient-care/measles/measles-frequently-asked-questions/#:~:text=100%20000%20IU%20 (30%20000,symptoms%20of%20vitamin%20A%20deficiency. Accessed April 7, 2025.

11. Rainwater-Lovett K, Moss WJ, Measles (rubeola), In: Loscalzo J, Kasper DL, Longo DL, et al, Harrison's Principles of internal medicine, 21st edition, 2025, McGraw-Hill, New York, 1607-1610. chapter 025. Available at: https://access medicine-mhmedical-com.proxy.libraries.rutgers.edu/content.aspx?sectionid= 265434623&bookid=3095&Resultclick=2 (Accessed 7 April 2025).

12. Centers for Disease Control and Prevention (CDC). About the vaccine: MMR and MMRV composition and dosage. 2021. Available at: https://www.cdc.gov/ vaccines/vpd/mmr/hcp/about.html#:~:text=M%2DM%2DR%20II%20and%20 PRIORIX%20are,%2C%20attenuated%20varicella%2Dzoster%20virus. Accessed April 7, 2025.

13. Centers for Dsiease Control and Prevention (CDC). Measles vaccine recommendations. 2024. Available at: https://www.cdc.gov/measles/hcp/vaccine-considerations/ index.html. Accessed April 7, 2025.

14. American Academy of Pediatrics. Measles. 2021. Available at: https://publications. aap.org/redbook/book/347/chapter-abstract/5753982/Measles?redirectedFrom= fulltext. Accessed April 7, 2025.

15. Centers for Disease Control and Prevention. Interim infection prevention and control recommendations for measles in healthcare settings. Available at: https:// www.cdc.gov/infection-control/hcp/measles/index.html. Accessed April 7, 2025.

Tick-Borne Infections in North America: An Overview

Mary DiGiulio, DNP, ANP-BC, GNP-BC[a],*,
Courtney Brown, MSN, ANP-BC[a,b]

KEYWORDS

- Tularemia • Tick-borne infection • Babesiosis • Ehrlichiosis • Anaplasmosis
- Lyme disease • Powassan virus • Rocky Mountain spotted fever

KEY POINTS

- Tick-borne infections range from asymptomatic to fatal diseases.
- Early identification and treatment are key to decreasing morbidity and mortality.
- Patient education on preventive strategies to avoid ticks is a major focus in controlling tick-borne disease.

INTRODUCTION

Tick-borne infections are a growing public health concern in North America as the incidence of some tick-borne diseases has doubled since 2000.[1] In the rest of the world, vector-borne diseases are primarily the result of mosquitoes; however, in the United States, ticks are the primary source of vector-borne illnesses.[2] The primary tick vectors affecting North America are *Ixodes scapularis*, *Amblyomma americanum*, *Dermacentor variabilis*, and *Ixodes pacificus*.[1,3] Tick vectors transmit viruses, bacteria, and protozoa with multiple illnesses sometimes transferred by one tick.[2] The most common tick-borne infectious disease in the United States and Canada is Lyme disease. **Fig. 1** shows the distribution of the more common tick-borne zoonotic infectious diseases in the United States.[4]

There are multiple risk factors for tick-borne diseases, some of which are modifiable.[1] Individuals who work outside or engage in a lot of outdoor activities including hiking, camping, and gardening are at higher risk of tick exposure and subsequently tick-borne illness.[1,3] Likewise, pet and livestock owners are at higher risk as well as migrant workers.[1] Tick-borne infections are more common from the months of April through October, which coincides with the peak of the tick populations and the season

[a] School of Nursing & Public Health, Moravian University, 1200 Main Street, Bethlehem, PA 18018, USA; [b] Graduate Nursing Faculty, Moravian University, Bethlehem, PA, USA
* Corresponding author. Moravian University, Helen S Breidegam School of Nursing and Public Health, 1200 Main Street, Bethlehem, PA 18018.
E-mail address: digiuliom@moravian.edu

Nurs Clin N Am 60 (2025) 431–447
https://doi.org/10.1016/j.cnur.2024.10.010
0029-6465/25/© 2024 Elsevier Inc. All rights reserved, including those for text and data mining, AI training, and similar technologies.
nursing.theclinics.com

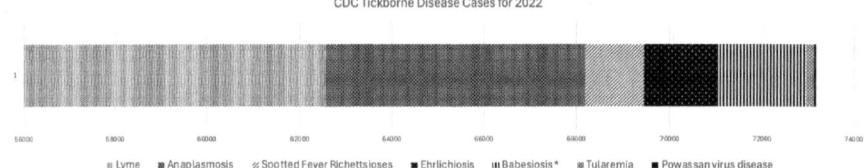

CDC Tickborne Disease Cases for 2022

☰ Lyme   ☰ Anaplasmosis   ⊠ Spotted Fever Richettsioses   ▪ Ehrlichiosis   ⅲ Babesiosis*   ⊠ Tularemia   ▪ Powassan virus disease

Fig. 1. CDC Tick-borne Disease CDC Tick-borne Disease Surveillance Data Summary. * denotes data is from 2021 as 2022 data was not available (only for Babesiosis). (*Source* Centers for Disease Control and Prevention. Tickborne Disease Surveillance Data Summary 2024. Accessed https://www.cdc.gov/ticks/data-research/facts-stats/tickborne-disease-surveillance-data-summary.html.)

humans are most likely to be outdoors.[2,3] Children aged between 5 and 14 years and adults aged between 55 and 79 years are at greater risk for tick-borne infections with male individuals having a greater risk than female individuals due to the time spent outdoors.[3]

Early identification and treatment is of utmost importance for full recovery.[3] Tick-borne infections are often difficult to diagnose due to the nonspecific symptoms seen in many instances. In addition, up to 50% of people diagnosed with a tick-borne disease do not recall a specific tick bite.[2] Testing is complicated as diagnostic tests vary depending on the phase of illness the patient is in at the time of testing.[2] The true incidence of tick-borne infections is not really known as some patients remain asymptomatic and the case identification and reporting requirements vary geographically.[3]

A potential solution to mitigate the tick population is through control of the habitat or use of acaricides; however, larger studies where this has been attempted have shown equivocal results leaving this as an area for further research.[5] Reducing tick exposure coupled with checking for ticks after outdoor activities remain the mainstay of prevention.[3]

TICK-BORNE ZOONOTIC DISEASES
Babesiosis

Introduction and background
Babesia is an intraerythrocytic and parasitic protozoan responsible for babesiosis.[5] It was first recognized in humans in 1957 in Europe; however, it was first described by Viktor Babes in 1888 when studying febrile cattle.[6] When considering tick-borne illnesses, babesiosis is of particular interest as rates of infection have increased over the past 20 years.[7] While babesiosis is most commonly transmitted through tick bites, there are cases of transfusion, organ transplantation, and placental transmission of babesiosis given the protozoal invasion of the erythrocyte.[3,6–8]

Epidemiology
Babesiosis is most commonly found in the Northeastern and Midwest of the United States with Massachusetts, Connecticut, Rhode Island, New York, New Jersey, Minnesota, and Wisconsin accounting for the majority of cases though there is expansion across the eastern US coast.[6] On average, there are 1910 cases in the United States per year, with approximately 6% to 23% of people concomitantly affected by Lyme given the overlap in vectors.[2,7] Cases in Canada have primarily been reported in Manitoba[3,9] and Ontario.[7] Rates of babesiosis are exponentially higher in the warmer months and when deer are in closer proximity to humans.[6] There may be coinfection with Lyme disease or anaplasmosis.[10]

Pathogenesis

There are multiple species of *Babesia* that can cause illness in humans; however, *Babesia microti* is by far the most common in the United States with *I scapularis* and *I pacificus* being the primary vectors.[7] There are ranges in the incubation period, with 1 to 4 weeks after tick attachment and 1 to 9 weeks after transmission via blood transfusion or organ transplantation.[11] After attachment occurs, the protozoa enters the capillaries and invades the erythrocytes where it grows and replicates.[12] After replication occurs, lysis of the erythrocyte takes place allowing the protozoa to invade new erythrocytes.[12] The majority of symptoms associated with *Babesia* infection is due to the lysis of the erythrocytes and subsequent proinflammatory cytokine release.[2,6]

Clinical presentation

For tick-borne infection of *B microti*, symptoms typically begin 1 to 4 weeks after transmission while transfusion-associated transmission can occur between 1 and 6 weeks[7] or between 1 and 9 weeks.[3] Approximately 25% of adult infections and 50% of pediatric infections are asymptomatic.[7] Those who develop symptoms most commonly have nonspecific complaints such as fevers, chills, and myalgias.[7] Examination findings include fever, organomegaly (spleen/liver), and splinter hemorrhages.[2] There may be nonspecific laboratory findings associated with *Babesia* infection including anemia, reticulocytosis, elevated lactic dehydrogenase (LDH), thrombocytopenia, transaminitis, proteinuria, and renal dysfunction.[2]

Patients who are immunocompromised or chronically ill can present with more severe symptomatology including organ failure, disseminated intravascular coagulation (DIC), and shock. More severe symptoms are usually associated with higher levels of parasitemia.[7,12] The fatality rate is between 2% and 9% in hospitalized cases with a fatality rate of up to 20% in transfusion-associated cases.[7]

Observation/assessment/evaluation

Giemsa staining is the gold standard for parasite detection of *Babesia*; however, when low levels of parasites are present, detection is difficult.[7] In addition, it takes a trained microscopist to properly detect parasitic infections. Serologic antibody testing is frequently difficult to interpret in the early stages of disease due to false-negative results.[2] Polymerase chain reaction (PCR) detection is relatively new but has significantly improved the diagnostic timeline and allows for testing with low parasitic counts.[6,12]

Management

Treatment of babesiosis involves an antiparasitic and an antibiotic. For mild-to-moderate disease, the treatment is atovaquone plus azithromycin.[7,13] For patients with severe disease, the treatment is quinine plus intravenous clindamycin[13] with some patients requiring an exchange transfusion.[7] The quinine plus clindamycin combination is not well tolerated, and there is documentation of babesiosis relapse in immunocompromised patients.[7]

Emerging therapies/emerging treatment

There are no current human vaccines. Potential vaccines may include whole parasite (inactivated or attenuated) vaccines and subunit vaccines utilizing surface antigens.[5,8]

Ehrlichiosis

Introduction and background

Ehrlichia chaffeensis is a gram-negative rickettsial coccobacillus responsible for the majority of ehrlichiosis cases in the United States.[12,14] This bacteria typically invades monocytes giving it the name of human monocytic ehrlichiosis or HME.[14] *E chaffeensis* was identified as a human vector in 1986 though *Ehrlichia* was taxonomically ranked in 1932.[7] *E chaffeensis* is a zoonotic organism with many vectors including domestic cattle and dogs contributing to its proliferation.[12] Due to the bacteria's invasion of monocytes, there are documented cases of infection secondary to organ transplantation and blood transfusions.[12]

Epidemiology
There are 3 to 5 per 100,000 cases of ehrlichiosis annually in endemic places with about 1377 cases reported per year.[7] While ehrlichiosis is found across the northeast, midwest,[7] mid-Atlantic,[7,15] southeast, south central US states,[15] approximately half of the cases in the United States are from the states of Missouri, Arkansas, North Carolina, and New York.[7,12]

Pathogenesis
E chaffeensis is primarily transmitted through the tick vectors of *A americanum*[3,7,16] and *D variabilis*,[7] it has also been found in *I scapularis*.[3,16] This organism is nonmotile and typically invades the phagosomes of monocytes so it can be found in many different body tissues and fluids.[7,12] Ehrlichiosis can be transmitted via blood or organ transplant.[16] The incubation period is approximately 1 to 2 weeks.[16] Bacteria can be found in the tick throughout the entire life cycle and is transmitted quickly after attachment making it very effective in transmission.[7] The symptoms of HME are thought to be secondary to the inflammatory response of the host.[2]

Clinical presentation
The symptoms of HME appear approximately 5 to 14 days after the tick bite occurs.[12] The primary symptoms are fever, chills, myalgia, headache, and gastroenterological symptoms such as nausea, vomiting, and diarrhea.[12] A maculopapular rash on the trunk or extremities develops in about a third of patients approximately 5 days after the onset of illness.[2,12,14] The rash occurs most commonly in children or immunocompromised adults.[12,14] Children can also present with edema while adults with severe infection may present with confusion, lymphadenomegaly,[12] uncontrolled bleeding, organ failure, and death.[16] Laboratory findings include transaminitis, leukopenia, and thrombocytopenia.[14] Approximately 60% of cases require hospitalization with the elderly and immunocompromised at higher risk for serious complications.[12] About 20% of patients have central nervous system (CNS) illnesses such as meningitis while 9% to 17% of cases result in serious complications such as organ failure.[7,14]

Observation/assessment/evaluation
The gold standard diagnostic test is culture; however, it is not frequently done due to the prolonged time to get results and the cost of the test.[7] The most common test done is serology as it is inexpensive and quick, but the provider must be aware that there are false negatives in the first week and periodically false positives.[12] Another option for diagnostics is a staining method; however, this is of limited use as it requires a highly trained microscopist.[7,12] PCR testing for DNA is best to use during the first week or so as it is widely available, sensitive, and specific.[7]

Management
As some of the aforementioned diagnostic tests have delays in confirming infection, it is recommended that patients who are symptomatic in endemic areas be treated empirically.[7] The treatment of choice for all ages is doxycycline typically for 5 to 7 days[16] though if there is Lyme coinfection 10 to 14 days is recommended.[7] In patients who cannot tolerate doxycycline, rifampin is used.[14]

Emerging therapies/emerging treatment
There are no current human vaccines.[16]

Lyme Disease

Introduction and background
Borrelia burgdorferi is a gram-negative spirochete bacteria responsible for Lyme disease, named after the town of Lyme, Connecticut, where it was first recognized in the 1970s.[17] Descriptions of a similar syndrome were published in Europe in the 1880s and antibiotics were prescribed for a similar syndrome in the 1940s.[7] Lyme disease is the most common tick-borne infection reported in Northern America,[17] Europe, Asia, and Russia. It is endemic in the northeast and northern midwest of the United States and eastern and central Canada.[7]

Lyme disease is transmitted via the I scapularis in the central and eastern United States and eastern and central Canada, and the I pacificus ticks in the western United States.[15,17] In 2016, Borrelia mayonii was also identified as a causative organism.

Epidemiology
The US Centers for Disease Control and Prevention (CDC)[18] received reports of 62,551 cases of Lyme disease in 2022, reflecting a 154% increase from reported cases in 2021. It was most commonly reported in New York, Pennsylvania, and New Jersey from 2015 through 2022.[18] In Canada, it is more commonly reported in the southern areas of Ontario, Manitoba, Quebec, and Nova Scotia.[3,19] Lyme disease is more likely to occur in the spring, summer, and fall months, with the highest incidence during the months of June and July, followed by August and May.[18] Transmission of Borrelia spirochetes is most common through the black-legged ticks: I scapularis, most commonly found in eastern and midwestern areas, and I pacificus, more common in western coast US states.[17] There may be coinfection with babesiosis or anaplasmosis.[10]

Pathogenesis
Infected ticks must be attached to the host for at least 24 hours to transmit the infecting organism.[20] Once the bacteria is transmitted to a human, there is an inflammatory response as the infecting organism multiplies and spreads locally while it evades the normal host immune response. The organism must first adapt to the host environment with its increased temperature, change in pH, and onslaught of innate immune response. As the spirochete replicates, it is able to penetrate the vasculature and enter the tissue matrix and colonize a variety of body tissues. Patients may experience manifestations involving the neurologic, cardiovascular, arthritic, and dermatologic systems as the spirochete binds to and colonizes varied tissues.[21] The incubation period from transmission to symptoms ranges from 3 to 30 days.[18]

Clinical presentation
Lyme disease is often described as having 3 stages—early localized, early disseminated, and late disease; however, the distinction among stages is not always clear.[17] The hallmark sign is erythema migrans, a nontender, nonitchy rash with a bullseye pattern that may feel warm to touch[17] is seen in up to 80% of patients.[20] Rashes may have an area of central clearing but also may not exhibit the classic bullseye appearance. Early symptoms include nonspecific flu-like symptoms of fever, chills, headache, myalgia, and arthralgia.[20]

Early presentation includes erythema migrans, fever, chills, headache, fatigue, and myalgia.[22] Later stages may overlap and may include multiple skin lesions, neurologic, cardiac, and arthritic involvement.[17] Neurologic involvement may include facial palsy (eg, Bell's palsy), meningitis, encephalopathy, and radiculopathy. Cardiac involvement may exhibit as Lyme carditis with myocarditis, atrioventricular heart block, and atrial fibrillation. Arthritic involvement may present as monoarticular or oligoarticular arthritis with joint swelling, a large effusion, and minor pain (disproportionate to the amount of swelling), most commonly affecting the knee.[17,23]

Observation/assessment/evaluation
Initially patients may present with fever, chills, headache, myalgia, arthritis, lymphadenomegaly, and erythema migrans. As the disease progresses, patients may have additional skin lesions, facial palsy, joint swelling that is more common in the knee or other large joints, myalgia, pain in tendons or bones, palpitations, irregular heart beat due to atrioventricular heart block, dizziness, shortness of breath, meningitis, or neuropathy.[20]

Two-step serologic testing for antibodies is recommended. In the first 4 to 6 weeks of infection, serologic testing may be falsely negative. The first step test is immunoassay followed by Western blot testing if the first test is positive or equivocal.[20]

Management
Recommended treatment of early localized disease in adults and children is with doxycycline OR amoxicillin or cefuroxime for up to 14 days. Consultation with infectious disease is appropriate for patients experiencing disseminated disease. For patients exhibiting neurologic symptoms, such as facial palsy, meningitis or radiculoneuritis, adults and children should be treated with doxycycline or ceftriaxone for 2 to 3 weeks. Treatment may be intravenously or oral, depending on patient condition. Lyme carditis with mild atrioventricular block should be treated with doxycycline OR amoxicillin OR cefuroxime for 2 to 3 weeks in adults and children. Patients experiencing more severe atrioventricular block should be treated with ceftriaxone for 2 to 3 weeks. Adults and children aged over 8 years experiencing arthritis should be treated with doxycycline, amoxicillin, or cefuroxime for 28 days. Children aged under 8 years should be treated with amoxicillin or cefuroxime for 28 days.[20]

For adults or children with an identified high-risk tick bite, prophylactic treatment may be indicated with single dose doxycycline within 72 hours of the bite.[24]

LYMErix was approved in 1998 as a vaccine for Lyme disease. Smith-Kline-Beecham (now Glaxo-Smith-Kline) voluntarily removed the vaccine in 2002. Efficacy of vaccine wanes over time, so those vaccinated prior to 2002 are no longer protected against Lyme disease.[20]

Emerging therapies/emerging treatment
Phase 3 clinical trials are underway for a multivalent, protein subunit Lyme vaccine.[20,25] (22-CDC Lyme Disease 2024, 26-Valneva) Monoclonal antibodies are being studied for use as pre-exposure prophylaxis at the start of the season for Lyme.[20]

Anaplasmosis

Introduction and background
Anaplasma phagocytophilum is a small, gram-negative rickettsial bacteria responsible for human granulocytic anaplasmosis (HGA) named so because of its invasion of granulocytic cells.[2] It was first identified as a pathogen in 1994 in North America, classified initially as part of the *Ehrlichia* species.[26] In 2001, it was renamed as *A phagocytophilum*, often referred to as anaplasmosis.[7] HGA is transmitted via *Ixodes* species of ticks; however, there are also documented cases of transmission secondary to blood transfusions.[10,12]

Epidemiology

There are approximately 4000 cases of anaplasmosis reported annually in the United States with June to November being the most common months of diagnosis.[7,12] Historically, this disease was seen in the northeastern and upper Midwest United States; however, there has been geographic expansion into Canada due to the proliferation of the *I scapularis* tick.[2,7] There may be coinfection with Lyme disease or anaplasmosis.[10]

Pathogenesis

A phagocytophilum is an intracellular bacteria that is transmitted from its primary reservoirs of the white-foot mouse and ruminants to humans via *Ixodes* ticks.[2,12] The bacteria invades granulocytes and multiples with the host response playing a large role in patient symptoms.[2] The incubation period is 1 to 2 weeks,[10] but it can extend to 21 days.[3]

Clinical presentation

Onset of symptoms is typically 5 to 14 days after tick bite with three-quarters of those infected recalling a recent tick bite.[2,7] Symptoms are generally self-limiting and include flu-like symptoms: fever, headache, myalgias, and in some cases gastrointestinal symptoms.[2] There are instances of more severe symptoms including bleeding, organ failure, and death, usually associated with patients who are immunocompromised or elderly.[10,12]

Observation/assessment/evaluation

Physical examination is usually unrevealing; however, laboratories may indicate leukopenia, thrombocytopenia, and transaminitis.[7] In the first 1 to 2 weeks, PCR testing is the most reliable; however, serologic testing is standard despite its limited use in the first 2 weeks of infection.[2]

Management

The recommendation is to start treatment if disease is suspected, do not wait for laboratory confirmation.[2] The treatment is doxycycline but rifampin is used if doxycycline is contraindicated.[2]

Emerging therapies/emerging treatment

There is no current vaccine available, but research is ongoing to develop one.[10]

Powassan

Introduction and background

Powassan encephalitis is caused by the Powassan virus, part of the *Flavivirus* genre.[7] Powassan was first discovered in humans in 1958 in Ontario.[8] The primary vectors are *I scapularis* and *Ixodes cookei*.[17] While this infection is uncommon, approximately half of those who are affected develop long-term neurologic complications making it a public health concern.[3]

Epidemiology

There are 133 cases of Powassan encephalitis documented annually in the United States, which is increasing though the reason is unclear.[7] The risk of Powassan is also low in Canada.[27] It may be secondary to increase in the *I scapularis* tick population, increased incidence, increased surveillance or some combination.[7,28] Distribution is primarily across the northeastern and northern Midwest United States.[7]

Pathogenesis

Powassan virus is a member of the *Flavivirus* genus family and is a single-stranded RNA, enveloped, dense virion that is surrounded by a lipid membrane.[29] Transmission from tick to host can occur in as little as 15 minutes, which is in contrast to other infections listed here that require longer attachment times.[14] The incubation period is 1 to 5 weeks.[30] In rare cases, the transmission of Powassan virus is possible through blood transfusion, and patients recovering from the illness should refrain from blood donation for at least 4 months.[30]

Clinical presentation
The initial presentation of Powassan virus is fever, headache, vomiting, and weakness, typically starting 1 to 4 weeks after infection.[3,30] This can progress to severe neurologic complications with headache, confusion, and neurologic deficits secondary to encephalitis and meningitis with a 10% to 15% mortality rate in these cases.[17,30] Long-term neurologic effects may include headaches, muscular weakness, focal paralysis, or cognitive impairment.[30]

Observation/assessment/evaluation
Serologic testing is the most common testing modality for Powassan virus. Testing may need to be performed at a state testing facility or the CDC. Testing may be done on serum or cerebrospinal fluid. Patients who test positive for Powassan-specific immunoglobulin (immunoglobulin M [IgM]) test should have a confirmatory plaque-reduction neutralization test at a state public health laboratory or at the CDC.[30]

Cerebrospinal fluid analysis may show neutrophils early in the disease and lymphocytic pleocytosis in patients with encephalitis or meningitis due to Powassan virus. Protein levels may be normal or slightly elevated and glucose level should be normal. Electroencephalogram will show slow wave activity in patients with Powassan virus encephalitis. MRI will show hyperintensities in superficial and deep white matter in patients with Powassan virus encephalitis.[30]

Management
There are no specific treatments available for Powassan infection and subjects' symptoms are treated supportively as they arise. Key to this disease is prevention given the lack of treatment options.[30]

Emerging therapies/emerging treatment
While there is no current vaccine for Powassan virus for humans, 4 different vaccine types are under development.[31]

Rocky Mountain Spotted Fever

Introduction and background
Rickettsia rickettsii is the bacteria responsible for Rocky Mountain spotted fever (RMSF).[32] RMSF has been a reportable disease since the 1920s,[4] and it is now one of several disorders that are collectively reported as spotted fever rickettsiosis.[32,33] RMSF is transmitted by *D variabilis*, *Dermacentor andersoni*, and *Rhipicephalus sanguineus*.[15,32] RMSF was first identified in Idaho in 1896.[34]

Epidemiology
D variabilis can be transmitted east of the Rocky Mountains, *D andersoni* can be transmitted in Rocky Mountain states and southwestern Canada at elevations of 4000 to 10,500 ft (approximately 1200–3200 m), and *R sanguineus* can be transmitted in the southwestern US and Mexico (33 - CDC Rocky Mountain Spotted Fever). RMSF can be transmitted throughout the contiguous United States, although more than half of cases are reported in North Carolina, Oklahoma, Arkansas, Tennessee, and Missouri.[15,32] The highest incidence is between May and August. The highest case fatality rates for spotted fever rickettsiosis are in those aged from 0 to 4 years then 5 to

9 years. This age group has a lower overall incidence, but a higher risk of fatality.[33] Transmission of RMSF by the R sanguineus tick in Arizona and northern parts of Mexico is more common near kennels or home settings, both indoors and outdoors and can occur year-round. These cases have a higher incidence and rate of fatality.[32]

Pathogenesis
RMSF progresses rapidly and can be fatal. Early treatment is needed to avoid death.[32] Providers need to consider RMSF in patients presenting with febrile illness as up to 10% of patients will not develop a rash and half will develop the rash within the first 3 days.[32] The incubation period is 3 to 12 days.[33]

Clinical presentation
The classic presentation includes fever, rash, and headache.[35] The rash typically develops 2 to 5 days after the onset of other symptoms, beginning on the limbs and spreading to the trunk and head.[33] The rash may spread to the palms and soles.[32] A macular rash may develop between days 2 and 4 with a petechial rash developing on day 5 or 6.[32] However, up to 10% of patients do not develop a rash despite having RMSF.[33]

Early symptoms occur during the first 4 days and include fever, headache, myalgia, malaise, periorbital edema, edema on the posterior surface of the hands, nausea, vomiting, and anorexia.[32,33]

Later symptoms include alterations in mental status, cerebral edema, pulmonary edema, acute respiratory distress syndrome, necrosis, and organ failure.[32] More severe illness can be seen in those who have a delay in treatment, children and those with glucose-6-phosphate dehydrogenase deficiency.[32]

Observation/assessment/evaluation
Antibody titers in the early stages of illness may be negative for up to a week to 10 days, and IgM antibodies are more likely to result in a false positive.[33] DNA may be detectable in a skin biopsy of a rash lesion or in whole blood during acute illness. Immunohistochemical staining can detect the bacteria in a biopsy specimen. PCR assays are available at certain laboratories.[33] Do not wait for laboratory confirmation if RMSF is suspected.

As the disease progresses, laboratory testing may also show thrombocytopenia, hyponatremia, and elevated hepatic transaminases.[32]

Management
Doxycycline is the drug of choice for all ages. Treatment duration is typically 5 to 7 days, or until 3 days after the fever subsides and other clinical symptoms improve.[33] Rapid desensitization is recommended for those with a significant allergy to doxycycline.[32]

Emerging therapies/emerging treatment
There is no vaccine to prevent RMSF.[32]

Tularemia

Introduction and background
Francisella tularensis is an aerobic, gram-negative coccobacillus that causes tularemia.[14] This disease is named after Tulare County, California where in 1911 it was isolated in squirrels, but it was subsequently discovered as a tick-borne illness in 1924.[2,36,37] Of note, tularemia is classified by the US Department of Health and Human Services as a List A agent for bioterrorism as it is not only a tick-borne illness,

but it is easily transmitted through other means such as close contact or aerosol transmission.[2]

Epidemiology
There are approximately 50 to 100 cases of tularemia in the United States per year with the *Ixodes* species of tick acting as vector.[14,37] Tularemia is clustered in the south central United States primarily in Oklahoma, Arkansas, Missouri, and Kansas.[2,14] While tularemia can be transmitted multiple ways, in the United States, the primary vectors are ticks and deer flies with ticks being the most common on the East Coast and flies being the most common west of the Rocky Mountains.[2,14] The most common time of transmission is between May and August as this is hunting season where humans spend exponentially more time in close proximity with nature.[36]

Pathogenesis
F tularensis enters the capillaries of the host after attachment by the vector. Once in the capillaries, it enters the macrophages where it replicates and then spreads to other macrophages primarily by direct cell-to-cell contact.[38] The incubation period is 3 to 5 days, but it can vary depending on the amount of bacteria that has been transmitted.[39]

Clinical presentation
There are multiple presentations of tularemia based on the mechanism of transmission, with tick-borne transmission presented primarily as ulceroglandular disease.[2] Patients develop flu-like symptoms 3 to 5 days after attachment with nonspecific symptoms including fever, headache, cough, and gastrointestinal symptoms.[2,14] A papule later develops that progresses into a painful, necrotic ulceration at the tick feeding site.[2,14,36] The patient will develop lymphadenopathy with fluctuance and sometimes drainage.[2,14]

Observation/assessment/evaluation
The preferred means for the diagnosis are bacterial cultures from a lymph node biopsy or purulent drainage from a lymph node.[14] Blood cultures, immunoassays, and serology testing can also be performed depending on the phase of illness.[14]

Management
Treatment of mild tularemia infection is tetracycline and ciprofloxacin.[2] Streptomycin or gentamicin can be used for more serious infections for 10 to 21 days.[14] Gentamicin and ciprofloxacin have been used successfully in treating tularemia, but are not Food and Drug Administration (FDA)-approved for this purpose.[40]

Emerging therapies/emerging treatment
Studies are ongoing to develop a vaccine for tularemia[41,42] (**Table 1**).

DISCUSSION

Providers should consider tick-borne illnesses in patients who live in or traveled to endemic areas presenting with an acute febrile illness with or without known exposure to ticks.[30] It is difficult to know the true burden of tick-borne infections as surveillance methods and reporting requirements vary by region. It is likely that the actual numbers of illnesses are underreported.[3] Early identification and treatment is critical for recovery and, in some cases, prevention of death or long-term complications.

Precautions for those engaging in outdoor activities, such as hiking, camping, scouting, occupational exposures should also be employed by those engaging in activities including gardening, golf, or walking the dog as animals (birds, deer, wild pigs,

Table 1
Tick-borne zoonotic infections in the United States and Canada

Disease	Tick	Organism (Type)	Incubation Period	Signs and Symptoms	Common Locations	Reportable	First-Line Treatment	Human Vaccine Available
Babesiosis	*I scapularis* (black-legged or deer tick), *I pacificus* (western black-legged tick)[16]	*B microti* most common in United States (Swanson 2023) *Babesia duncani* and *Babesia divergens*[3] (parasite)	1–4 wk after tick bite; 1–9 wk following blood products or solid organs[11]	Asymptomatic to severe disease and death; fevers, chills, myalgias, headache,[7] gastrointestinal (GI) symptoms; respiratory distress, hemolytic anemia, reticulocytosis, thrombocytopenia, splinter hemorrhages, elevated LDH, transaminitis, proteinuria, organomegaly, organ failure, disseminated intravascular coagulation, and death[2,8] Increased risk of life-threatening illness in those with comorbidities, immunocompromise, infants and adults aged over 50 years[3]	United States— northeast and midwest Canada—Ontario[3,43] Manitoba[3,9]	United States— Yes in 40 states[13] US blood donations screened in 14 states and DC[9] Yes—Canada 2024 to present[44]	Asymptomatic— no treatment needed for most Symptomatic with mild-to-moderate symptoms in outpatient setting treat orally atovaquone *with* azithromycin OR clindamycin *with* quinine For moderate-to-severe symptoms in hospitalized patient threat with oral atovaquone *with* IV azithromycin OR IV clindamycin *with* oral quinine[13]	No[8]
Human monocytotropic ehrlichiosis	*A americanum* (lone star tick),[3,7,15,16] *D variabilis osis* 2024) *D variabilis* (American dog tick) (Madison Antonucci)	*E chaffeensis* (bacteria)	1–2 wk[16]	Fever, myalgia, headache, N/V/ D,[3] (maculopapular or petechial rash (more common in children)[16] children—edema; adults with severe infection— lymphadenomegaly, confusion,[12] meningoencephalitis, organ failure, bleeding, and death[16]	United States— black-legged tick: upper midwest, eastern, Lone star tick—eastern, southeast, south central states[15] Canada— unknown	United States— Yes[7,16] Canada—No[3]	Doxycycline for adults and children[15]	No[15]

(continued on next page)

Table 1
(continued)

Disease	Tick	Organism (Type)	Incubation Period	Signs and Symptoms	Common Locations	Reportable	First-Line Treatment	Human Vaccine Available
	I scapularis (black-legged tick) (CDC where ticks live)							
Lyme	I scapularis (black-legged or deer tick), I pacificus (western black-legged tick)[15,17]	B burgdorferi, B mayonii[21] (spirochete bacteria)	3–30 d[23]	Early—include fever, chills, headache, myalgia, arthralgia, and erythema migrans[17,20] Later—cardiac (myocarditis, atrioventricular heart block, atrial fibrillation), neurologic (Bell's palsy, meningitis, encephalopathy, and radiculopathy), arthritis (monoarticular or oligoarticular) with large effusion[17,23]	United States—Northeast, mid-Atlantic, upper midwest[23] Canada—All provinces with highest concentrations in Manitoba, Ontario, Quebec, and Nova Scotia[3,19]	United States—Yes[7] Canada—Yes[3] 2009–present[44]	Early disease—adults and children: doxycycline OR amoxicillin OR cefuroxime for up to 14 d Neurologic symptoms—adults and children: doxycycline or ceftriaxone for 2–3 wk Lyme carditis with mild heart block—adults and children: doxycycline OR amoxicillin OR cefuroxime for 2–3 wk Lyme carditis with more severe heart block—adults and children: ceftriaxone for 2–3 wk Arthritis in adults and children aged 8+ years:	No Clinical trials underway for vaccine[25] The vaccine LYMErix by Smith-Kline-Beecham was US FDA approved in 1998 but was voluntarily removed from the market in 2002[20]

Disease	Tick vector	Pathogen	Incubation	Symptoms	Geographic distribution	Established	Treatment	Prophylaxis
							doxycycline, amoxicillin, or cefuroxime for 28 d; Arthritis in children aged <8 y: amoxicillin or cefuroxime[20]; Postexposure prophylaxis for adults and children within 72 h of high-risk tick bite—single dose doxycycline[24]	
Anaplasmosis	I scapularis (black-legged or deer tick), I pacificus (western black-legged tick)[15]	A phagocytophilum (bacteria)	1–2 wk[7], 5–21 d[3]	Initially—flu-like symptoms: fever, headache, myalgias, possible GI symptoms;[2] more severe symptoms including bleeding, organ failure, and death[10,12]	United States—Northeast and upper midwest; Canada—all provinces with increased incidence in Ontario.[43]	United States—Yes[10]; Yes—Canada 2024–present[44]	Doxycycline; Rifampin if doxycycline contraindicated2	No[10]
Powassan	I scapularis (black-legged or deer tick)[15]; Ixodes spinipalpis[3]	Powassan virus, deer tick virus[30] (virus)	1–5 wk[30]	Initial—fever, headache, vomiting, and weakness; Severe disease—encephalitis, meningitis[30]	United States—northeastern and northern Midwest United States[7]; Manitoba	United States—Yes[30]; Canada—Yes 2024–present[44]	Supportive care[30]	No[31]

(continued on next page)

Table 1
(continued)

Disease	Tick	Organism (Type)	Incubation Period	Signs and Symptoms	Common Locations	Reportable	First-Line Treatment	Human Vaccine Available
					Canada—Ontario, Quebec, Manitoba, Atlantic Provinces, Nova Scotia, British Columbia, and New Brunswick[27]			
*Rocky Mountain spotted fever**	*D variabilis* (American dog tick) *D andersoni* (Rocky Mountain wood tick) *R sanguineus* (brown dog tick)[15,32]	*R rickettsii*[15] (bacteria)	3–12 d[33]	Classically—fever, rash, and headache (King 2024) Rash absent in up to 10% of patients (CDC Tickborne diseases of the US) Early symptoms—Fever, headache, rash, nausea, vomiting, abdominal pain, myalgia, and anorexia[32] Later symptoms—change in mental status, cerebral edema, pulmonary edema, acute respiratory distress syndrome, necrosis, organ failure, and potentially fatal[32]	United States—contiguous US states[32] Canada—southwestern Canada from 4000 to 10,500 ft elevation[32]	United States—Yes[4] Canada—1930–1978[44]	Doxycycline[32]	No[32]
Tularemia	*D andersoni* (Rocky Mountain wood tick), *D variabilis* (American dog tick), *A americanum* (lone star tick)[14,15,37]	*Francisella tularensis*[14] (bacteria)	3–5 d[39]	Flu-like symptoms (fever, headache, cough, and GI symptoms) followed by a papule that evolves into a painful necrotic ulceration[2,14,36]	United State—south, central US[2,14] Canada—Rare[41]	United State—Yes[40] Canada—Yes[41]	Mild—tetracycline and ciprofloxacin[2] Streptomycin or gentamicin can be used for more serious infections for 10–21 d[14]	Under development[42]

hedgehogs, and mice) are often found in suburban outdoor spaces as natural habitats are destroyed.[1]

Geographic areas of tick populations are expanding and may be contributed to global warming, animal migration, urbanization, or deforestation.[3] Further study on impact of climate change on geographic distribution of ticks and tick-borne illness.[17]

SUMMARY

Patients should be instructed in ways to avoid ticks to reduce potential exposure to tick-borne illnesses. Use of personal protective measures such as wearing loose, light colored clothing, tucking in clothing at the waist and ankles, using approved repellents appropriate for the patient's age, and removing clothing worn outdoors and checking for ticks once back inside. Permethrin-treated clothes are appropriate for adults. Clothing worn outdoors can be laundered or placed in the dryer on high heat prior to next wearing.[3]

Tick-borne infections have seasonal trends with the majority of cases reported during warmer weather in the spring, summer, and fall. Providers should have increased awareness of the possibility of tick-borne illnesses in those living in or near endemic areas.[3] Asking patients about outdoor activities and recent travel can aid in identification of potential tick-borne illnesses.

CLINICS CARE POINTS

- Early identification and treatment is important for full recovery.
- Patients may not recall tick bite.
- Neonates, older patients, those with immune compromise or significant comorbidities are at an increased risk of sever disease or death.
- Treatment options may be limited in pregnancy and breastfeeding.[3]
- Patient education on risk of tick-borne illness and methods to reduce tick exposure are necessary.[1]

REFERENCES

1. Kim P, Maxwell S, Parijat N, et al. Targeted tick-borne disease recognition: assessing risk for improved public health. Healthcare 2024;12(10):984.
2. Eilbert W, Matela A. Tick-borne diseases. Emerg Med Clin North Am 2024;42(2):287–302.
3. Elmieh N, National Collaborating Centre for Environmental Health (NCCEH). A review of health risks associated with tick exposure for Canadians. Vancouver, BC: NCCEH; 2022. Available at: https://ncceh.ca/resources/evidence-reviews/review-ticks-canada-and-health-risks-exposure. Accessed October 7, 2024.
4. Centers for Disease Control and Prevention. Tickborne disease surveillance Data summary. 2024. Available at: https://www.cdc.gov/ticks/data-research/facts-stats/tickborne-disease-surveillance-data-summary.html. Accessed October 1, 2024.
5. Diakou A. Biting back: advances in fighting ticks and understanding tick-borne pathogens. Pathogens 2024;13(1):73.
6. Vannier EG, Diuk-Wasser MA, Ben Mamoun C, et al. Babesiosis. Infect Dis Clin North Am 2015;29(2):357–70.

7. Madison-Antenucci S, Kramer LD, Gebhardt LL, et al. Emerging tick-borne diseases. Clin Microbiol Rev 2020;33. https://doi.org/10.1128/cmr.00083-18.

8. Jerzak M, Gandurski A, Tokaj M, et al. Advances in *Babesia* vaccine development: an Overview. Pathogens 2023;12(2):300.

9. Swanson M, Pickrel A, Williamson J, et al. Trends in reported babesiosis cases — United States, 2011–2019. MMWR Morb Mortal Wkly Rep 2023;72:273–7.

10. Centers for Disease Control and Prevention. Anaplasmosis. 2024. Available at: https://www.cdc.gov/anaplasmosis/site.html#gen. Accessed October 8, 2024.

11. Public Health Agency of Canada. National case definition: babesiosis. 2024. Available at: https://www.canada.ca/en/public-health/services/diseases/babesiosis/health-professionals/national-case-definition.html. Accessed October 9, 2024.

12. Andonova R, Bashchobanov D, Gadzhovska V, et al. Tick-borne diseases—still a challenge: a review. Biologics 2024;4(2):130–42.

13. Centers for Disease Control and Prevention. Babesiosis. 2024. Available at: https://www.cdc.gov/babesiosis/about/index.html. Accessed October 8, 2024.

14. Rodino KG, Theel ES, Pritt BS. Tick-borne diseases in the United States. Clin Chem 2020;66(4):537–48.

15. Centers for Disease Control and Prevention. Where ticks live. 2024. Available at: https://www.cdc.gov/ticks/about/where-ticks-live.html. Accessed October 1, 2024.

16. Centers for Disease Control and Prevention. Ehrlichiosis. 2024. Available at: https://www.cdc.gov/ehrlichiosis/about/index.html. Accessed October 1, 2024.

17. Sullivan MD, Glose K, Sward D. Tick-borne illnesses in emergency and wilderness medicine. Emerg Med Clin North Am 2024;42(3):597–611.

18. Centers for Disease Control and Prevention. Lyme disease surveillance Data. 2024. Available at: https://www.cdc.gov/lyme/data-research/facts-stats/surveillance-data-1.html. Accessed September 28, 2024.

19. Public health agency of Canada Lyme disease: monitoring. 2024. Available at: https://www.canada.ca/en/public-health/services/diseases/lyme-disease/surveillance-lyme-disease.html. Accessed October 10, 2024.

20. Centers for Disease Control and Prevention. Lyme disease. 2024. Available at: https://www.cdc.gov/lyme/index.html. Accessed September 29, 2024.

21. Coburn J, Garcia B, Hu LT, et al. Lyme disease pathogenesis. Curr Issues Mol Biol 2021;42:473–518.

22. Watts J, Taylor K. Gentrification increases risk of tick-borne disease for communities of colour. Nat Microbiol 2024;9:312–3.

23. Centers for Disease Control and Prevention. Yellow book Lyme. 2024. Available at: https://wwwnc.cdc.gov/travel/yellowbook/2024/infections-diseases/lyme-disease. Accessed September 30, 2024.

24. Lantos PM. AAN/ACR/IDSA 2020 guidelines for the prevention, diagnosis and treatment of Lyme disease. Clin Infect Dis 2021;72(1):e1–48.

25. Valneva. Pfizer adn valnexa complete recruitment for phase 3 VALOR trial for Lyme disease vaccine candidate, VLA15. 2023. Available at: https://valneva.com/press-release/pfizer-and-valneva-complete-recruitment-for-phase-3-valor-trial-for-lyme-disease-vaccine-candidate-vla15/. Accessed October 10, 2024.

26. Schudel S, Gygax L, Kositz C, et al. Human granulocytotropic anaplasmosis—a systematic review and analysis of the literature. PLoS Neglected Trop Dis 2024;18(8):e0012313. Available at: https://journals.plos.org/plosntds/article?id=10.1371/journal.pntd.0012313. Accessed September 29, 2024.

27. Public Health Agency of Canada. Powassan virus disease. 2024. Available at: https://www.canada.ca/en/public-health/services/diseases/powassan-virus/risks.html.

28. Hermance ME, Thangamani S. Powassan virus: an emerging arbovirus of public health concern in NorthNorth America. Vector Borne Zoonotic Dis 2017;17(7): 453–62.

29. Kemenesi G, Bányai K. Tick-borne flaviviruses, with a focus on powassan virus. Clin Microbiol Rev 2018;32. https://doi.org/10.1128/cmr.00106-17.

30. Centers for Disease Control and Prevention. Powassan virus. 2024. Available at: https://www.cdc.gov/powassan/about/index.html. Accessed October 1, 2024.

31. Cheung AM, Yip EZ, Ashbrook AW, et al. Characterization of live-attenuated powassan virus vaccine candidates identifies an efficacious prime-boost strategy for mitigating powassan virus disease in a murine model. Vaccines (Basel) 2023; 11(3):612. Available at: https://pmc.ncbi.nlm.nih.gov/articles/PMC10058527/. Accessed October 10, 2024.

32. Centers for Disease Control and Prevention. Rocky Mountain Spotted Fever. 2024. Available at: https://cdc.gov/rocky-mountain-spotted-fever/about/index.html (Accessed 10 October 2024).

33. Centers for Disease Control and Prevention. Tick borne diseases of the US. 2022. Available at: https://www.cdc.gov/ticks/hcp/data-research/tickborne-disease-reference-guide/?CDC_AAref_Val=https://www.cdc.gov/ticks/tickbornediseases/index.html. Accessed October 7, 2024.

34. National Institute of Health. National institute of allergy and infectious diseases, . Rocky Mountain spotted fever. Available at: https://www.cdc.gov/anaplasmosis/site.html#gen.

35. King A, Spurr A, Bose R. Rocky Mountain spotted fever contracted along a Canadian road trip: a case report. SAGE Open Med Case Rep 2024;12. https://doi.org/10.1177/2050313X241260980. 2050313X241260980.

36. Troha K, Božanić Urbančič N, Korva M, et al. Vector-borne tularemia: a Re-emerging cause of cervical lymphadenopathy. Tropical Medicine and Infectious Disease 2022;7(8):189.

37. Yeni DK, Büyük F, Ashraf A, et al. *Tularemia:* a re-emerging tick-borne infectious disease. Folia Microbiol 2021;66:1–14.

38. Degabriel M, Valeva S, Boisset S, et al. Pathogenicity and virulence of *Francisella tularensis.* Virulence 2023;14(1). https://doi.org/10.1080/21505594.2023.2274638.

39. European Centre for Disease Prevention and Control. Tularemia. 2024. Available at: https://www.ecdc.europa.eu/en/tularaemia. Accessed October 11, 2024.

40. Centers for Disease Control and Prevention. Tularemia. 2024. Available at: https://www.cdc.gov/anaplasmosis/site.html#gen. Accessed October 11, 2024.

41. National Collaborating Centre for Infectious Diseases. Francisella tularensis (tularemia disease). Available at: https://nccid.ca/debrief/francisella-tularensis-tularemia-disease/. Accessed October 11, 2024.

42. Harrell JE, Roy CJ, Gunn JS, et al. Current vaccine strategies and novel approaches to combatting Francisella infection. Vaccine 2024;42(9):2171–80.

43. Public health Ontario ENHANCED EPIDEMIOLOGICAL SUMMARY anaplasmosis and babesiosis in Ontario: 2023. 2024. Available at: https://www.cdc.gov/anaplasmosis/site.html#gen. Accessed October 9, 2024.

44. Public Health Agency of Canada. Case definitions: nationally notifiable diseases. Available at: https://diseases.canada.ca/notifiable/diseases-list.

Norovirus Infection

A Clinical Overview for Nurses and Nurse Practitioners

Jeffrey Kwong, DNP, MPH, AGPCNP-BC*

KEYWORDS

- Norovirus • Gastroenteritis • Dehydration • Diarrheal outbreaks

KEY POINTS

- Norovirus is one of the leading causes of infectious gastroenteritis globally.
- Although infection with norovirus is self-limited, some patients are at greater risk for morbidity, including pediatric and older adult populations, as well as those who are immunocompromised.
- Nurses play a key role in early recognition and educating patients on management and prevention of disease.

CASE VIGNETTE

A 72 year old man with a past medical history of hypertension, hyperlipidemia, prediabetes, and osteoarthritis presents to the emergency room with complaints of 3 days of persistent, nonbloody diarrhea and weakness. He believes his symptoms started shortly after eating raw oysters at a local restaurant. The patient reports having 10 to 12 loose, watery bowel movements per day. Other associated symptoms include feeling feverish, weakness, nausea, and abdominal bloating. He has been trying to keep hydrated but is afraid to eat anything because that will trigger his need to go to the bathroom. On physical examination, his temperature is 101.2°F, blood pressure is 110/76 mm Hg, his pulse is 110 beats per minute, respirations are 16 breaths per minute, and his oxygen saturation is 96% on room air. Orthostatic blood pressure readings were obtained and demonstrated a drop in diastolic blood pressure of greater than 10 mm Hg after standing with an increase in his heart rate. He appears fatigued. His mucous membranes are dry. His cardiopulmonary examination is normal. He has hyperactive bowel sounds. There are no abdominal masses, but he

Division of Advanced Nursing Practice, Rutgers School of Nursing, Newark, NJ, USA
* Corresponding author. 65 Bergen Street, Newark, NJ 07107.
E-mail address: Jeffrey.Kwong@Rutgers.Edu
Twitter: @jkwong_np (J.K.)
Instagram: nurse_jeff_nyc

Nurs Clin N Am 60 (2025) 449–454
https://doi.org/10.1016/j.cnur.2024.11.002   **nursing.theclinics.com**
0029-6465/25/© 2024 Elsevier Inc. All rights reserved, including those for text and data mining, AI training, and similar technologies.

has some diffuse right and left lower quadrant tenderness with palpation. There is no guarding or rebound tenderness. The patient is given a 500 cc bolus of 0.9% normal saline. Laboratory studies were obtained. His creatinine was 1.3 mg/dL, blood urea nitrogen (BUN) was 20 mg/dL, potassium was 3.4 mmol/L, sodium was 135 mmol/L, and glucose was 68 mg/dL. The patient was admitted with dehydration secondary to gastroenteritis. Stool studies were obtained. His *Clostridioides difficile* antigen and giardia antigen were negative. A polymerase chain reaction (PCR) gastrointestinal pathogen panel was positive for norovirus.

INTRODUCTION

Infectious gastroenteritis is one of the more common infectious diseases globally, affecting an estimated 685 million annually.[1] Although most of these infections are self-limiting, some individuals can experience significant morbidity that can lead to acute complications of dehydration, metabolic derangement, and in severe cases death. Nurses should be familiar with the care and management of persons with infectious gastroenteritis. This article will review the epidemiology, pathophysiology, clinical presentation, diagnosis, and management of persons with norovirus. Strategies for prevention and infection control will also be reviewed.

EPIDEMIOLOGY

According to the Centers for Disease Control and Prevention, norovirus is the leading pathogen of infectious gastroenteritis in the United States and is associated with over 2.2 million outpatient clinic visits, 465,000 emergency department visits, 109,000 hospitalizations, and 900 deaths.[1] While the majority of emergency visits and office visits are in young children, the number of deaths is typically among those aged older than 65 years. Given that norovirus is associated with foodborne illnesses, data show that norovirus accounts for 58% of all reportable foodborne illness cases.[1] Globally, the incidence of norovirus infection is estimated to be 685 million cases annually. One-third of the global cases (200 million) occur in children aged under 5 years, of which 50,000 pediatric cases result in mortality.[1]

Throughout the United States, localized outbreaks of norovirus occur each year. Most recent data indicate that there are about 2500 reported outbreaks annually.[1] Although norovirus infections can occur at any time throughout the year, historically in the United States there is a rise in cases between November and April.[2] An outbreak is cluster of 2 or more cases stemming from a common source. Outbreaks of norovirus have been seen in a variety of settings and among different populations. Common settings that have been reported in the past include health care facilities, long-term care, cruise ships, restaurants, schools, childcare facilities, college and universities, and military units.[1,3,4]

The economic burden of norovirus infection is also notable. Norovirus is estimated to cost US$2 billion in health-related expenditures in the United States, and US$60 billion globally.[5] These costs are inclusive of the cost of direct care as well as lost productivity. Analysis of the health care burden of norovirus globally suggests that the majority costs are due to lost productivity and that the economic impact of norovirus exceeds that of other enteric viruses.[5]

PATHOPHYSIOLOGY

Norovirus is a nonenveloped, positive-sense RNA virus that is part of the Caliciviridae family of viruses. The first cases of norovirus are believed to date back to the 1929 when individuals would experience what was termed, "winter vomiting disease."[6] Subsequently in 1968, an outbreak among school-aged children in Norwalk, Connecticut led to the initial identification of norovirus (which at that time was given the name Norwalk virus). It was not until 1972 that the prototype strain was officially identified.[6] Current understanding of norovirus reveals that there are multiple different strains and variants of the virus that can causes illness.

The exact mechanism in which norovirus causes disease in humans is uncertain. There have been several theories regarding pathogenesis of disease. One theory suggests that microfold cells (or M cells), which are a special type of enterocyte in the gut lumen, transport the virus to the host's underlying immune cells in the intestinal tract causing disease.[7] Other theories suggest that there might be an interaction between the host's gut microbiome and commensal bacteria, which may facilitate infection.[7]

The typical incubation period for disease is 12 to 48 hours after infection.[8] Norovirus is highly virulent and requires little inoculum to cause disease. Some reports suggest that as few as 10 virions may be sufficient to cause disease in humans, which contributes to the ease and rapidity of outbreaks.[9]

TRANSMISSION

Norovirus is spread primary through fecal–oral transmission.[1] This can occur from person-to-person when one individual is infected with norovirus, through contaminated food and water (eating food that has been in contact with contaminated water or eating raw fruits and vegetables that have not been washed), as well as through surfaces that have been inoculated with the virus. Norovirus has the ability to live on environmental surfaces and be transmitted to others by this route. More recent studies indicate the possibility of aerosolization of the virus, especially in persons with norovirus who are vomiting.[10] Persons coming into close contact with someone with norovirus who is vomiting may be at risk for inhalation of aerosolized particles that may lead to infection. Additionally, data have shown that in persons who have recovered from the symptomatic period of infection can still shed norovirus for weeks to even months after resolution of symptoms.[11]

CLINICAL PRESENTATION

The most common symptoms of norovirus infection include acute onset of nausea, vomiting, diarrhea, abdominal pain, fever, and chills. Individuals who may experience dehydration secondary to volume loss from diarrhea, may also experience dizziness, headache, and weakness.[12]

As part of the patient history, nurses should inquire about symptom onset and duration. Inquire about consumption of any new foods or foods known to be associated with norovirus infection—including raw seafood such as oysters. Any exposure to persons with similar symptoms or recent known norovirus infection is also important to ascertain. Travel and occupational history can also assist in identifying potential risk factors for infection. Physical examination findings may include hypotension, tachycardia, dry mucous membranes, and decreased skin turgor.

DIAGNOSIS AND LABORATORY TESTING

The diagnosis of norovirus is made primarily on history and physical examination. Laboratory testing is not required for diagnosis. However, if testing is needed or performed, norovirus can be detected on real time PCR stool pathogen panels.[12] In patients who may have dehydration, a comprehensive metabolic panel is useful to assess for any renal, electrolyte, or hepatic abnormalities. Based on history and consideration for other causes of acute diarrhea, additional stool studies may be warranted to help confirm the diagnosis, including stool culture, ova and parasites, and testing for *C difficile*.[13]

MANAGEMENT

The mean duration of illness is 2 days in most healthy individuals. Prolonged symptoms can be seen in young children, older adults, or those who may be immunocompromised. Treatment and management of infection is focused on symptomatic care and hydration. Use of empiric antibiotics is not recommended. For pediatric patients, the use of oral rehydration solutions with glucose and electrolytes is recommended over sports drinks because sports drinks may increase diarrheal symptoms due to the high carbohydrate and osmotic load.[13]

For adults with irretractable nausea, use of antiemetics, such as ondansetron, can be used. For pediatric patients, antiemetics are not recommended, except in mild-to-moderate dehydration when nausea interferes with oral rehydration therapy.[13] Eating small meals that are bland and low residue may also be helpful. Antimotility agents are not recommended, especially in pediatric patients.[12,13]

PREVENTION

One of most effective form of prevention is hand washing with soap and water.[14] Norovirus is not killed by alcohol-based sanitizers. Educate and inform individuals to carefully wash fruits and vegetables. Individuals who are sick or recently recovered should avoid preparing food or meals for others.

If caring for someone who is vomiting or who has diarrhea, providers should use standard and contact precautions.[15] Be sure to wear gloves and a disposable gown. Given the possibility of aerosolization in persons who are vomiting, a mask and eye protection can help reduce the possibility of transmission or unintended splashes. In the inpatient setting, patients should be placed in single occupancy rooms and movement of patients out of rooms should be minimized.[15]

Disinfect and wipe all surfaces in patient care areas with health care grade disinfectants. For patients with norovirus who are cared for at home, a bleach solution with a concentration of 1000 to 5000 ppm (5–25 tablespoons of household bleach [5%–8% per gallon of water]) can be used to clean environmental surfaces at home to prevent transmission to others.[14] Linens and clothes that are soiled with feces or vomit should also be laundered and cleaned immediately.

At this time, there is no vaccine for norovirus, although clinical trials investigating preventive vaccines have been developed. Various vaccine strategies, including oral, injectable, intradermal, and intranasal vaccines are being studied.[16]

FOLLOW-UP

As previously stated, most cases of norovirus are self-limiting, and patients recover without any significant complications. Long-term follow-up is typically not required. Patients with norovirus infection are susceptible to reinfection; therefore, patient education on ways to minimize reinfection is critical.

SUMMARY

Infectious gastroenteritis is one of the leading infections that nurses in the acute and ambulatory care settings will encounter as part of routine practice. Given the virulence and morbidity associated with norovirus infection, it is important to have early recognition of the illness to help treat patients appropriately and, more importantly, avoid or limit the spread of this viral infection to others. From a public health perspective, norovirus infection has been associated with regional outbreaks and remains one of the infections that is monitored on a regular basis by local and federal public health officials. Nurses play a critical role in providing supportive care for patients who are ill and educating patients, family members, and the community on ways to reduce the risk of transmission to help control and contain this virus, which has impacted communities across the globe.

CLINICS CARE POINTS

- Patients with signs or symptoms of infectious gastroenteritis should be assessed for dehydration.
- Symptomatic patients with evidence of severe dehydration or who are at risk for complications associated with dehydration should be assessed for the need for intravenous hydration and admission.
- If norovirus is suspected or confirmed with diagnostic testing, patients should be placed on contact precautions if hospitalized. If patients are managed at home, all members of the household should wash hands with soap and water frequently, especially after using the bathroom, and to limit contact as much as possible.
- Individuals with norovirus infection should avoid preparing food for others for at least 48 hours after symptoms subside.

DISCLOSURE

The author has nothing to disclose.

REFERENCES

1. Centers for Disease Control and Prevention (CDC), Norovirus facts and stats, Available at: https://www.cdc.gov/norovirus/data-research/index.html#:~:text =Norovirusworldwide,childrenunder5yearsold (Accessed 18 November 2024), 2024.
2. Grytdal S, Browne H, Collins N, et al. Trends in incidence of norovirus-associated acute gastroenteritis in 4 veterans affairs medical center populations in the United States, 2011-2015. Clin Infect Dis 2020;70(1):40–8.
3. Calderwood LE, Wikswo ME, Mattison CP, et al. Norovirus outbreaks in long-term care facilities in the United States, 2009-2018: a decade of surveillance. Clin Infect Dis 2022;74(1):113–9.
4. Queiros-Reis L, Lopes-João A, Mesquita JR, et al. Norovirus gastroenteritis outbreaks in military units: a systematic review. BMJ Mil Health 2021;167(1):59–62.
5. Bartsch SM, Lopman BA, Ozawa S, et al. Global economic burden of norovirus gastroenteritis. PLoS One 2016;11(4):e0151219.
6. Lucero Y, Matson DO, Ashkenazi S, et al. Norovirus: facts and reflections from past, present, and future. Viruses 2021;13(12):2399.
7. Karst SM, Tibbetts SA. Recent advances in understanding norovirus pathogenesis. J Med Virol 2016;88(11):1837–43.

8. Centers for Disease Control and Prevention (CDC), About norovirus, Available at: https://www.cdc.gov/norovirus/about/index.html (Accessed 18 November 2024), 2024.

9. Teunis PF, Moe CL, Liu P, et al. Norwalk virus: how infectious is it? J Med Virol 2008;80(8):1468–76.

10. Tan M, Tian Y, Zhang D, et al. Aerosol transmission of norovirus. Viruses 2024; 16(1):151.

11. Qiu Y, Freedman SB, Williamson-Urquhart S, et al. Significantly longer shedding of norovirus compared to rotavirus and adenovirus in children with acute gastro-enteritis. Viruses 2023;15(7):1541.

12. Capece G. and Gignac E., Norovirus, Available at: https://www.ncbi.nlm.nih.gov/books/NBK513265/#:~:text=Onceadiagnosisofnorovirus,keepupdatedo nhygieniccodes (Accessed 18 November 2024), 2024.

13. O'Ryan M.G., Norovirus, Available at: https://www.uptodate.com/contents/norovirus (Accessed 18 November 2024), 2024.

14. Centers for Disease Control and Prevention (CDC), How to prevent norovirus, Available at: https://www.cdc.gov/norovirus/prevention/index.html (Accessed 18 November 2024), 2024.

15. Centers for Disease Control and Prevention (CDC), Infection control summary and recommendations, Available at: https://www.cdc.gov/infection-control/hcp/norovirus-guidelines/summary-recommendations.html (Accessed 18 November 2024), 2024.

16. Cortes-Penfield NW, Ramani S, Estes MK, et al. Prospects and challenges in the development of a norovirus vaccine. Clin Therapeut 2017;39(8):1537–49.

The Right Drug for the Bug

Prescribing Antibiotics in an Era of Resistance by Using Antibiograms to Inform Decision Making

Teri Moser Woo, PhD, ARNP, CPNP-PC[a,b]

KEYWORDS

- Antibiotic resistance • Antibiogram • Antibiotic prescribing

KEY POINTS

- More than 39 million people worldwide may die in the next 25 years from antimicrobial-resistant infections.
- Antibiotic resistance for multiple pathogens increased during the COVID pandemic.
- Bacteria, fungi, and viruses can develop resistance to antimicrobials by developing protective mechanisms or sharing genetic material with other pathogens.
- Guidelines provide recommendations for first-line antibiotic choices. Using an antibiogram will allow the prescriber to tailor the antibiotic choice based on local resistance patterns.

INTRODUCTION

According to a recent systematic analysis, it is estimated that more than 39 million people worldwide may die in the next 25 years from antimicrobial-resistant infections.[1] Up to 2 million deaths annually may be directly attributed to antimicrobial resistance and 8.22 million deaths will possibly be associated with antimicrobial resistance in 2050, with the greatest burden among those age 70 years of age or older.[1] To mitigate the high number of forecasted deaths, a combination of infection prevention, immunizations, research into new antibiotics, and minimizing inappropriate antibiotic prescribing will be needed.

The focus of this review is to discuss how antimicrobial resistance in the United States impacts prescribing decisions. Pathogens impacting health due to increasing resistance will be reviewed. How pathogens develop resistance and share genetic elements across pathogens leading to resistance that impacts prescribing will be discussed. Guidelines-based empiric prescribing and antibiograms to guide rational

[a] Pediatric ARNP, Mary Bridge Children's Pediatric Urgent Care, 1700 5th Street Southeast, Suite 100, Puyallup, WA 98372, USA; [b] HRSA Nursing Workforce Diversity grant, Saint Martin's University, Lacey, WA, USA
E-mail address: twoo@stmartin.edu

Nurs Clin N Am 60 (2025) 455–464
https://doi.org/10.1016/j.cnur.2024.10.008
0029-6465/25/© 2024 Elsevier Inc. All rights reserved, including those for text and data mining, AI training, and similar technologies.

prescribing will be examined to decrease inappropriate broad-spectrum antibiotic prescribing.

ANTIBIOTIC RESISTANCE THREATS

The US Centers for Disease Control and Prevention (CDC) is responsible for monitoring existing and emerging antibiotic resistance in the United States. In 2013, the CDC published the first *Antibiotic Resistance (AR) Threats*, updated in 2019 to include 18 antimicrobial-resistant bacteria and fungi.[2] The pathogens in the 2019 *AR Threats* report are categorized into 3 categories based on the impact on human health: urgent, serious, and concerning. The 2019 report also included a "watch list" of 3 pathogens that are of concern for developing significant resistance (**Table 1**). Among the urgent threats is *Candida auris* (*C auris*), a multidrug-resistant candida that can cause life-threatening infections in ill or immunocompromised patients and is highly communicable in health care facilities. *C auris* was first identified in the United States in 2013 and experienced a 5-fold increase between 2019 and 2022 during the COVID pandemic.[3] *Neisseria gonorrhoeae* is also identified as an urgent threat due to the fact it has developed resistance to all classes of antibiotics except for ceftriaxone, with ciprofloxacin no longer recommended and cefixime not recommended as the first-line treatment.[4] Enterobacteriaceae (including *Escherichia coli* and *Klebsiella pneumoniae*) can develop resistance to carbapenem and broad-spectrum beta-lactam antibiotics and thus is high on the list of antibiotic threats.[2]

In 2024, the CDC published updated data on 7 AR pathogens of concern specifically in health care settings.[3] During the COVID-19 pandemic, resistance increased for 6 of the 7 pathogens for a combined 20% increase in resistance, with only methicillin-resistant *Staphylococcus aureus* (MRSA) remaining stable (**Fig. 1**).[3] In 2025, the CDC is updating the estimates for 19 pathogens electronically to guide work to fight antibiotic resistance and to serve as a resource for clinicians.

HOW ANTIBIOTICS DEVELOP RESISTANCE

I don't work in the hospital or care for patients with gonorrhea, so I do not have to worry about those pathogens in my patients.

Understanding how antibiotic resistance develops and spreads is critical to prevent contributing to further resistance by inappropriate prescribing. Bacteria develop resistance by exposure to antibiotics leading to the development of defense mechanisms and by sharing genetic elements.[5,6] When pathogens are exposed to antibiotics, they evolve to develop resistance mechanisms including drug inactivation, limiting drug uptake, altering the drug target, and drug efflux.[6,7] Antibiotics may be deactivated or neutralized by enzymes produced by the pathogen, as seen in B-lactamase production which attacks the B-lactam ring in the B-lactam antibiotics.[7] Bacteria are able to alter or remodel their outer membrane making it more difficult for antibiotics to penetrate the bacteria. Bacteria can also alter the targets of the antibiotics including lipid A modification, ribosomal alteration, and RNA methylation.[5–7] Efflux pumps can actively transport the antibiotic out of the cell.[6,7] Another avenue in which bacteria develop resistance is by sharing mobile genetic elements by transduction (transferring genes from one pathogen to another), conjugation (resistant genes transferred between pathogens when they connect), and transformation (resistant genes are released from nearby live or dead pathogens and picked up by another pathogen).[6,7] In practical terms, this means that bacteria can genetically share resistance to an antibiotic that is overprescribed such as azithromycin or ciprofloxacin.

Table 1
2019 Centers for Disease Control and Prevention antibiotic resistance threats

Pathogen	Comments
Urgent Threats	
Carbapenem-resistant *Acinetobacter*	Pneumonia and wound, bloodstream, and urinary tract infections. Tend to occur in patients in intensive care units (ICUs)
Candida auris (C auris)	Multidrug-resistant candida. Outbreaks in health care facilities.
Clostridioides difficile (C difficile)	May cause life-threatening diarrhea. Most often in people who have taken antibiotics
Carbapenem-resistant Enterobacteriaceae (CRE)	CRE include *Escherichia coli* and *Klebsiella pneumoniae.* Up to 30% of CRE can carry a mobile genetic element that produces an enzyme that makes carbapenem antibiotics ineffective and spread resistance
Neisseria gonorrhoeae	Gonorrhea easily develops resistance, and half of all infections are resistant to at least one antibiotic. Third-generation cephalosporins (ceftriaxone) are the only drug class without significant resistance.
Serious Threats	
Campylobacter	Causes diarrhea (often bloody), fever, abdominal cramps from raw or undercooked chicken, unpasteurized milk, contaminated food and water, and through direct contact with animals.
Drug-resistant *Candida* species	Cause candida infection including oral and vaginal infections. May also cause invasive *Candida* infections
Extended-spectrum beta-lactamase (ESBL) producing Enterobacteriaceae	The Enterobacteriaceae family includes *Escherichia coli,* and are common community-acquired AR infections
Vancomycin-resistant Enterococci (CRE)	Usually health care-associated exposures including long-term care, ICUs, cancer therapy, and organ transplant
Multidrug resistant *Pseudomonas aeruginosa (P aeruginosa)*	Health care-associated infections
Drug-resistant nontyphoidal *Salmonella*	Diarrhea (sometimes bloody), fever, and abdominal cramps from eating contaminated food or contact with infected animals
Salmonella typhi	Often associated with travel to countries where typhoid is common and is 74% resistant to ciprofloxacin. Vaccination before travel may prevent infection.
Shigella	Can cause diarrhea, fever, abdominal pain
Methicillin-resistant *Staphylococcus aureus* (MRSA)	Health care and community-acquired staph infections
Drug-resistant *Streptococcus pneumoniae* (pneumococcus)	The leading cause of bacterial pneumonia and meningitis in the United States. Decreasing with increased immunization with pneumococcal vaccine.

(*continued on next page*)

Table 1 (continued)	
Pathogen	Comments
Drug-resistant tuberculosis	Multidrug-resistant (MDR) TB is resistant to 2 first-line antibiotics. Extensive drug-resistant (XDR) TB is resistant to some first-line and second-line antibiotics.
Concerning Threats	
Erythromycin-resistant Group A *Streptococcus* (GAS)	Up to 35% of GAS is resistant to erythromycin. Azithromycin has cross-resistance to erythromycin-resistant *Streptococcus* isolates.
Clindamycin-resistant Group B *Streptococcus* (GBS)	Causes bloodstream infections, pneumonia, meningitis, and skin infections—in people of all ages including maternal transmission of GBS during labor and delivery to infants.
Watch List	
Azole-resistant *Aspergillus fumigatus* (*A fumigatus*)	The leading cause of invasive mold infections in humans
Drug-resistant *Mycoplasma genitalium*	Sexually transmitted infection which causes symptomatic and asymptomatic urethritis among men, and cervicitis, pelvic inflammatory disease in women. Azithromycin resistance is rapidly increasing.
Drug-resistant *Bordetella pertussis*	Growing macrolide resistance in Vietnam and China

Abbreviations: AR, antibiotic resistance; CDC, Centers for Disease Control and Prevention.
Data from: Center for Disease Control and Prevention (2019). Antibiotic Resistance Threats in the United States, 2019. Center for Disease Control. Atlanta, GA, U.S. Department of Health and Human Services.

RATIONAL PRESCRIBING OF ANTIMICROBIALS
Guidelines-Based Prescribing

In practice, most antibiotic prescribing is initially empiric based on the medical diagnosis (ie, pneumonia, otitis media, urinary tract infection [UTI]) and guidelines regarding first-line antibiotic recommendations. Guidelines are developed by experts and incorporate resistance patterns in recommending first-line antibiotic therapy, which is why guidelines for first-line therapy may change with updates. Updated guidelines for most infectious diseases or diseases that require antibiotic treatment are listed on the Infectious Diseases Society of America (IDSA) Web site (https://www.idsociety.org/), as well as professional society Web sites. The IDSA provides Clinical Practice Guidelines which are based on a systematic review of available evidence and evidence-based recommendations, as well as clinical guidance based on comprehensive review and clinical experts which are not graded. The CDC summarizes antibiotic prescribing guidelines for common infectious diseases seen in adult and pediatric practice reviewing the epidemiology, diagnostic criteria, and disease management (https://www.cdc.gov/antibiotic-use/hcp/clinical-care/). The CDC also provides updated guidelines for treating sexually transmitted diseases (www.cdc.gov/sti). There are several evidence-based mobile apps available for providers to utilize in decision-making when prescribing antibiotics (**Table 2**).

Prescribing Based on Antibiograms of Local Resistance Patterns

While national guidelines are helpful, it is also important to understand local antibiotic resistance patterns, which are found in local antibiograms. An antibiogram utilizes

Threat	Change in Rates or Number of Infections[c]			
	2020 vs. 2019	2021 vs. 2020	2022 vs. 2021	2022 vs. 2019
URGENT[a] Hospital-onset CRE	▲ Increase	▲ Increase	▬ Stable	▲ Increase
Hospital-onset Carbapenem-resistant *Acinetobacter*	▬ Stable	▬ Stable	▬ Stable	▲ Increase[b]
Clinical Cases of *C. auris*	▲ Increase	▲ Increase	▲ Increase	▲ Increase
SERIOUS[a] Hospital-onset MRSA	▲ Increase	▬ Stable	▼ Decrease	▬ Stable
Hospital-onset VRE	▲ Increase	▲ Increase	▬ Stable	▲ Increase
Hospital-onset ESBL-producing Enterobacterales	▲ Increase	▬ Stable	▬ Stable	▲ Increase
Hospital-onset MDR *Pseudomonas aeruginosa*	▲ Increase	▲ Increase	▬ Stable	▲ Increase

Fig. 1. Antimicrobial resistance threats in the US table shows change in rates and number of infections from 2019 to 2022. [a]Threat level for each pathogen, as categorized in CDC's antibiotic resistance threats in the United States, 2019. [b]There was no statistically significant difference in rate of hospital-onset carbapenem-resistant Acinetobacter in 2020, 2021, and 2022 when compared with the previous year. However, there was a statistically significant increase in rate of hospital-onset carbapenem-resistant Acinetobacter in 2022 when compared with 2019. [c]Hospital-onset rates were described using multivariable models for all threats except *C auris*. Please note that in above table, stable indicates there was no statistically significant increase or decrease, decrease indicates a statistically decrease where $P<.05$, and increase indicates statistically significant increase where $P<.05$ for all threats except for *C auris*. Increases or decrease in *C auris* was indicated by changes in the number of clinical cases reported nationally without hypothesis testing. (*From*: Centers for Disease Control (2024). "Antimicrobial Resistance Threats in the United States, 2021-2022." Retrieved 10/1/24 from https://www.cdc.gov/antimicrobial-resistance/data-research/threats/update-2022.html.)

Table 2 Antibiotic prescribing apps	
Source	**Contents**
CDC STI Treatment Guide Mobile App	Streamlined STI prevention, diagnostic, and treatment recommendations (free)
First Line	Health system-specific guideline recommendations incorporating local resistance patterns. Subscription product based on health care organization participation. Canadian and WHO guidelines included.
Infectious Diseases Society of America (IDSA) Practice Guidelines App	Latest guidelines and interactive point-of-care tools (free)
John Hopkins Antibiotic Guide	Subscription product, includes monthly updates, webinars, and comments from infectious disease and pharmacy experts
Sanford Guide Mobile App	Subscription product includes all the content from the print edition

Abbreviations: CDC, Centers for Disease Control and Prevention; STI, sexually transmitted infection; WHO, World Health Organization.

microbiologic data from local patient specimens. Antibiograms may be developed by a health care facility, health system, or local government such as the county or state health department. The Clinical and Laboratory Standards Institute (CLSI) has guidelines for the development and publication of antibiograms, which include annual updates.[8] An antibiogram is usually presented as a chart with the gram-positive and gram-negative pathogens listed on one axis and the pathogens on another axis with the susceptibility to specific antibiotics in the table (**Fig. 2**). When selecting an antibiotic to empirically treat an infection, the provider should select an antibiotic with the highest susceptibility appropriate for the site of the infection and suspected pathogen.[9] Examples of how to utilize an antibiogram in clinical practice are included here.

Case Studies Using Antibiograms

Child with a urinary tract infection

An 18-month-old female presents with a fever of up to 102°F for 4 days, fussiness, decreased appetite but good fluid intake, and no vomiting. A cathed point-of-care urinalysis indicated 3+ leukocytes, 1+ protein, and 2+ blood. The urine has been sent for culture. What would be the first-line antibiotic choice?

This case is an example of understanding the guidelines and utilizing local resistance patterns. The American Academy of Pediatrics (AAP) guideline for treating febrile UTI in children 2 months to 2 years of age recommends oral treatment of UTIs in children able to tolerate oral antibiotics to include a cephalosporin, amoxicillin plus clavulanic acid, or trimethoprim-sulfamethoxazole.[10] The AAP guidelines note it is important to know local resistance patterns when choosing an antibiotic for the initial treatment of a UTI as there is significant variation in susceptibility to antibiotics, particularly trimethoprim-sulfamethoxazole and cephalexin.[10] It is critical to understand the disease pathology, as using only antibiogram data may lead the provider to choose nitrofurantoin to treat the child's UTI, yet nitrofurantoin does not achieve parenchymal and serum concentrations and will not treat pyelonephritis or urosepsis.[9,10] Once the

Gram (-)	# of patients	Aminoglycosides			B-Lactams			Cephalosporins				Quinolones		Others
		Amikacin	Gentamikin	Tobramycin	Ampicillin	Imipenem	Piperacillin Tazobactam	Cefzolin	Cefoxitin	Ceftriaxone	Ceftazidime	Ciprofloxacin	Nitrofurantoin	TMP/SMX
Escherichia coli	4	100	100	100		100	100					100	75	
Klebsiella sp	13	100	84.6	92.3	38.5	100	92.3	84.6	100	100	100	38.5	92.3	38.5
Proteus sp	7	71.4	57.1	71.4		85.7	85.7			57.1	57.1	28.6		71.4
Pseudomonas aeruginosa	13	100	83.3	92.3	91.7		100			81.8	100	100	30.8		69.2

Gram (-)	# of patients	Penicillins				Cephalosporins		Quinolones		Others						
		Penicillins	Ampicillin	Oxacillin	Nafcillin	Cephalothin	Ceftriaxone	Ciprofloxacin	Moxifloxacin	Gentamicin	Linezolid	Rifampin	Tetracycline	TMP/SMX	Vancomycin	Nitrofurantoin
Staph aureus (all)	8	0		0	0			0	0	87.5	100	100	100	100	100	100
Methicillin Resistant (MRSA)	8	0		0	0			0		87.5	100	100	100	100	100	100
Methicillin Susceptible (MRSA)	0															
Enterococcus sp	4	100	100					50		75			25		100	100

Fig. 2. Example of an antibiogram. (*From*: Agency for Healthcare Research and Quality (2014). "Concise Antibiogram Toolkit." Retrieved 10/1/24 from https://www.ahrq.gov/sites/default/files/wysiwyg/professionals/quality-patient-safety/patient-safety-resources/resources/nh-asp guide/module2/toolkit1/cat_sources.pdf.)

urine culture is available, the provider has susceptibility data specific to the child's infection and can change the antibiotic if the pathogen is resistant to the initial antibiotic choice.

Adult with an abscess

A young adult with no history of a previous MRSA abscess presents with an abscess on their upper leg that is 1 cm in diameter with mild surrounding erythema. An incision and drainage of the abscess is completed, and the purulent drainage is sent for culture. Due to the size of the abscess and surrounding mild cellulitis, an antibiotic is indicated. What would be the first-line antibiotic choice?

The IDSA guidelines for the treatment of skin and soft tissue infections are dated, and new guidelines are prioritized for the development by IDSA. The IDSA guidelines developed in 2014 provide an algorithm for treating skin and soft tissue infections, including abscesses.[11] The IDSA guidelines recommend incision and drainage of the abscess and treating moderate or severe abscesses with trimethoprim/sulfamethoxazole (TMP/SMX), doxycycline, dicloxacillin, or cephalexin.[11] S aureus may exhibit different resistance patterns based on geography, with the highest percentage of MRSA isolates in the Southern United States.[12] Therefore, when choosing an empiric treatment for an abscess while awaiting culture results, a local antibiogram should be consulted to select an appropriate initial antibiotic with the most susceptibility to S aureus, the most likely pathogen in a simple abscess. Culture results with antibiotic sensitivity will confirm whether the chosen antibiotic provides coverage for the pathogen.

Diabetic foot ulcer

A 38-year-old with diabetes presents with a mild infection of the great toe. The patient is afebrile, has had no recent hospitalizations, and has no known risk for MRSA. Purulent drainage from the infected site has been sent for culture. What would be the empiric treatment for this patient?

The IDSA in collaboration with the International Working Group on the Diabetic Foot (IWGDF) has guidelines on the diagnosis and treatment of diabetes-related foot infections.[13] The IWGDF/IDSA guidelines recommend treating mild soft tissue foot infections with antibiotics that target gram-positive pathogens (beta-hemolytic streptococci and S aureus), with the first-line empiric therapy for uncomplicated mild infection cloxacillin or a first-generation cephalosporin (cephalexin).[13] The guidelines outline treatment for patients with B-lactam allergy as clindamycin; fluoroquinolone (levofloxacin/moxifloxacin); trimethoprim-sulfamethoxazole; or doxycycline; and if MRSA is suspected treat with linezolid; trimethoprim-sulfamethoxazole; clindamycin; doxycycline, or a fluoroquinolone (levofloxacin, moxifloxacin).[13] When choosing among antibiotics for empiric treatment, using an antibiogram to evaluate local resistance patterns will assist in choosing the best antibiotic for empiric treatment.

Positive strep test in a patient with "penicillin allergy"

A 17-year-old presents to urgent care with a sore throat, temperature of 102°F, swollen tonsillar lymph nodes, and nausea. Their immunizations are up-to-date. Their parent states "We don't give them amoxicillin because they got a rash when they were a baby when they took amoxicillin." A point-of-care strep tests positive for Group A strep. What would be the appropriate antibiotic to prescribe?

The CDC provides guidelines for the treatment of Group A streptococcal pharyngitis.[14] The first-line treatment for Group A strep pharyngitis is penicillin or amoxicillin. In this case, the parents report a rash with amoxicillin, therefore, an antibiotic choice for a patient with possible penicillin allergy would be cephalexin, cefadroxil, clindamycin, azithromycin, or clarithromycin.[14] While there has never been documented Group

Table 3
Strategies advanced practice nurses can use in practice

Strategy	Rationale	Recommendation
Avoid prescribing antibiotics for viral respiratory illness	When patients are prescribed an antibiotic such as azithromycin on day 3 of a URI or for "bronchitis" it is not only inappropriate prescribing but sets a precedent for patients to then ask for a Z-pack with every cough or cold. We need to save the use of azithromycin for pertussis and chlamydia which do not have good alternative treatments	Follow guidelines for diagnosing and managing viral respiratory infections, sinusitis, and acute uncomplicated bronchitis.
Use the most narrow-spectrum antibiotic indicated for the condition	Inappropriate use of broad-spectrum antibiotics leads to increased resistance.	Utilize a local antibiogram for empiric prescribing targeting the suspected pathogen with the appropriate antibiotic. "The right drug for the bug"
Reconsider prescribing fluconazole as first-line for symptoms of vaginitis or thrush	Overuse of fluconazole for vaginal candida infections or infants with thrush has led to fluconazole-resistant candida species, complicating treatment when serious systemic candida infections occur.	Use oral nystatin for infants with thrush. Follow CDC STI guidelines for the treatment of uncomplicated vulvovaginal candidiasis which is OTC topical azole antifungals (clotrimazole, miconazole, tioconazole) as first-line treatment
Accurately document penicillin allergy in medical record	Only true Type I allergic responses (hives, angioedema, wheezing, etc.) should be recorded as an allergy. Too often any rash is documented as penicillin allergy when "amoxicillin rash" is known to occur in ~ 5% of patients taking amoxicillin and is not a true hypersensitivity reaction. Inappropriate listing of penicillin/amoxicillin as an allergy leads to prescribing of broader spectrum antibiotics which increases resistance.	Follow CDC recommendations and only list Type I responses as an allergy in the medical record. The CDC recommends allergy testing which includes an oral challenge to rule out penicillin allergy.
Utilize a local antibiogram when choosing empiric antibiotic treatment	Antibiotic susceptibility can vary regionally and using a local antibiogram will inform empiric prescribing and will target local resistance patterns.	Local antibiograms can be found at the health system, laboratory, or county level. Some state health departments list the antibiograms available for their state.

Abbreviations: CDC, Centers for Disease Control and Prevention; OTC, over the counter; STI, Sexually transmitted infection; URI, upper respiratory tract infection.

A streptococcus resistance to penicillin or cephalosporins, there is significant (up to 35%) resistance to azithromycin, clarithromycin, and clindamycin which varies geographically.[14,15] Utilizing a local antibiogram will guide in choosing whether to treat with cephalexin, azithromycin, or clindamycin. New guidelines for treating strep pharyngitis are in development and are expected to be published in *Clinical Infectious Diseases* in late 2024 or early 2025.

Regarding the "rash" after taking amoxicillin described by the parents in the case study, the CDC has developed extensive resources regarding the overdiagnosis of penicillin allergy, noting that 10% of US patients report a penicillin allergy, but less than 1% are truly allergic.[16] When the patient has a penicillin allergy on their medical record broad-spectrum antibiotics are often used, leading to increased risk for antimicrobial resistance. The CDC recommends reviewing the patient's history and physical examination and only recording an immunoglobulin E-mediated (Type I) reaction to penicillin in the medical record as an allergy.[16] The CDC also recommends allergy testing to determine if a patient is truly allergic to penicillin.[16]

SUMMARY

Antibiotic resistance is a serious health threat predicted to increase over the next 25 years. Every antibiotic prescription written can contribute to resistance by the pathogen developing protective mechanisms or sharing genetic material with other pathogens, therefore, each antibiotic prescribed should be narrowly targeted to the suspected pathogen and inappropriate antibiotics avoided (**Table 3**). Using guidelines and referring to a local antibiogram when empirically prescribing antibiotics will improve patient outcomes and slow the growth of antibiotic resistance related to inappropriate prescribing.

CLINICS CARE POINTS

- Review your personal antibiotic prescribing patterns for over or inappropriate prescribing.
- Seek out your local antibiogram to understand local resistance patterns.
- Resist pressure to prescribe for known viral infections such as a URI or bronchitis.

REFERENCES

1. GBD 2021 Antimicrobial Resistance Collaborators. Global burden of bacterial antimicrobial resistance 1990-2021: a systematic analysis with forecasts to 2050. Lancet 2024;404(10459):1199–226.
2. Center for Disease Control. Antibiotic resistance threats in the United States, 2019. Alanta, GA: U.S. Department of Health and Human Services; 2019.
3. Centers for disease control and prevention. Antimicrobial resistance threats in the United States, 2021-2022. U.S. Department of health. Available at: https://www.cdc.gov/antimicrobial-resistance/data-research/threats/update-2022.html. Accessed October 1, 2024.
4. Center for Disease Control and Prevention. Sexually transmitted infections treatment guidelines, 2021. US Centers for Disease Control Updated; 2021. Available at: https://www.cdc.gov/std/treatment-guidelines/. Accessed September 30, 2024.
5. Zahari NIN, Engku Abd Rahman ENS, Irekeola AA, et al. A review of the resistance mechanisms for β-lactams, macrolides and fluoroquinolones among

streptococcus pneumoniae. Medicina (Kaunas) 2023;59(11). https://doi.org/10.3390/medicina59111927.

6. Centers for disease control and prevention. About antimicrobial resistance. U.S. Department of Health, Available at: https://www.cdc.gov/antimicrobial-resistance/about/index.html (Accessed 30 September 2024).

7. Gauba A, Rahman KM. Evaluation of antibiotic resistance mechanisms in gram-negative bacteria. Antibiotics (Basel) 2023;12(11). https://doi.org/10.3390/antibiotics 12111590.

8. Clinical and Laboratory Standards Institute. 5th edition. Analysis and presentation of cumulative antimicrobial susceptibility test data, 152. Malvern, PA: Clinical and Laboratory Standards Institute; 2022.

9. Truong WR, Hidayat L, Bolaris MA, et al. The antibiogram: key considerations for its development and utilization. JAC Antimicrob Resist 2021;3(2):dlab060.

10. Roberts KB, Subcommittee on Urinary Tract Infection SCoQI, Management. Urinary tract infection: clinical practice guideline for the diagnosis and management of the initial UTI in febrile infants and children 2 to 24 months. Pediatrics 2011; 128(3):595–610.

11. Stevens DL, Bisno AL, Chambers HF, et al. Practice guidelines for the diagnosis and management of skin and soft tissue infections: 2014 update by the Infectious Diseases Society of America. Clin Infect Dis 2014;59(2):e10–52.

12. Carrel M, Smith M, Shi Q, et al. Antimicrobial resistance patterns of outpatient staphylococcus aureus isolates. JAMA Netw Open 2024;7(6):e2417199.

13. Senneville É, Albalawi Z, van Asten SA, et al. IWGDF/IDSA guidelines on the diagnosis and treatment of diabetes-related foot infections (IWGDF/IDSA 2023). Clin Infect Dis 2023. https://doi.org/10.1093/cid/ciad527.

14. Center for Disease Control and Prevention. Clinical guidance for Group A streptococcal pharyngitis. U.S. Centers for Disease Control Updated; 2024. Available at: https://www.cdc.gov/group-a-strep/hcp/clinical-guidance/strep-throat.html#cdc_generic_section_8-treatment. Accessed September 26, 2024.

15. Center for disease control and prevention. ABCs bact facts interactive data dashboard. U.S. Centers for Disease control. 2024. Available at: https://www.cdc.gov/abcs/bact-facts/data-dashboard.html. Accessed September 27, 2024.

16. Center for Disease Control and Prevention. Clinical features of penicillin allergy. U.S. Centers for Disease control. 2024. Available at: https://www.cdc.gov/antibiotic-use/hcp/clinical-signs/index.html. Accessed September 2, 2024.

Hospital-Acquired Infections in the Elderly
Prevention Strategies

Amita Avadhani, PhD, DNP, NEA-BC, CNE, DCC, ACNP-BC, AGNP-C, CCRN, FCCM, FNAP[a],*, Joelle D. Hargraves, DNP, MSN, RN, CCRN, CCNS[b], Michael McIntosh, PhD, RN, CIC[c], Bernadette Sheeron, DNP, AGACNP-BC, ANP-BC[b]

KEYWORDS

- Infections • Hospital-acquired • Elderly • Prevention strategies

KEY POINTS

- Elderly patients are at high risk of hospital-acquired infections (HAIs) and worse morbidity and mortality outcomes.
- HAIs are preventable through source control and clean hands.
- Hospitals need to develop a culture of infection prevention.

INTRODUCTION

Hospital-acquired infections (HAIs) account for over 140,000 deaths per year and cost the US health care system over $14.9 billion annually.[1,2] There has been a dramatic increase in the number of HAIs and antibiotic-resistant infections since the coronavirus disease (COVID) pandemic.[3] These antibiotic-resistant strains are becoming more resistant and deadly. Some of the most common hospital acquired infections (HAI) pathogens include methicillin-resistant *Staphylococcus aureus* (MRSA), vancomycin-resistant enterococci (VRE), Acinetobacter, Klebsiella, *Escherichia coli*, Enterobacter, and *Clostridium difficile* infection (CDI).[4] These pathogens can be shed from infected or colonized patients and live on surfaces for long periods of time, up to several months.[5] Elderly patients are vulnerable for developing infections as they have a higher likelihood of having multiple comorbidities, a weakened immune system, and declining functional status; this risk increases if hospitalization occurs.[3] In addition to their risk

[a] Department of Nursing, College of Public Health, Temple University, 1316 Ontario Street (Jones Hall), Room 502, 3307 Broad Street, Philadelphia, PA 19140, USA; [b] College of Public Health, Temple University, 1316 Ontario Street (Jones Hall), Room 502, Philadelphia, PA 19140, USA; [c] Manager Infection Prevention - Ambulatory, Cooper University Health Care, 1 Cooper Plaza, Camden, NJ 08103, USA
* Corresponding author. Temple University Health Science Campus, Nursing Department-College of Public Health, 3307 North Broad Street, Jones Hall, Room 502, Philadelphia, PA 19140.
E-mail address: amita.avadhani@temple.edu

Nurs Clin N Am 60 (2025) 465–477
https://doi.org/10.1016/j.cnur.2024.10.006
nursing.theclinics.com
0029-6465/25/© 2024 Elsevier Inc. All rights reserved, including those for text and data mining, AI training, and similar technologies.

factors, the elderly are more likely to use medical equipment when hospitalized.[2] The most common types of infections related to medical equipment include central-line-associated bloodstream infection (CLABSI), catheter-associated urinary tract infection (CAUTI), and ventilator-associated events (VAEs).[5] These infections generally occur 48 hours after admission and are defined as HAIs. HAIs are a major threat to the safety of our patients, particularly our elderly.

HAIs pose a major global health and public health threats in individuals aged 65 years or older, with unfavorable health outcomes.[6–13] The complex interplay among biologic, pathogenic, social, and health care factors among individuals aged 65 years and older increases the incidence and prevalence of HAIs.[7,14,15] These factors coupled with noncommunicable diseases, decreases in socioeconomic stability, and poor dietary intake further elevate the incidence and prevalence of HAIs in this population age group.[13–15] Studies reporting factors influencing HAIs on the individuals aged 65 years and older are limited in their statistical and epidemiologic scope.[6] What is known is that the risk of contracting HAIs in individuals aged 65 years or older increases linearly with age.

The epidemiologic data are replete on HAIs in individuals aged 65 years and older. However, when available, the statistical and epidemiologic data are generalized, scattered, and incomplete.[6–11] HAIs are infections that occur in individuals while receiving care in a health care facility, including acute care hospitals (ACHs), long-term care (LTC) facilities (longtern care facilities [LTCFs]), outpatient surgical centers, dialysis, and ambulatory care centers.[13,16–24] Individuals aged 65 years and older are likely to reside in LTCFs, giving them increased exposure to chronic in-dwelling urinary catheters, feeding tubes, and central line or peripheral venous catheters, respiratory devices (eg, ventilators), and elevated potential for colonization of multidrug-resistant organisms (MDROs).[13,16–24] Alanazi and colleagues found that the health care delivery processes and attitudes of health care professionals toward safety and quality of health care delivery contribute to HAIs, especially in individuals aged 65 years and older.[19]

A study by Emori and colleagues[21] that examined data from the National Nosocomial Infections Surveillance System collected between 1986 and 1990 found that over half of all HAIs in the United States occurred in individuals aged 65 years and older. Tesini and Dumyati[22] found that urinary tract infections (UTIs) were the most common HAI in individuals aged 65 years or older, accounting for 44% of all infections, followed by pneumonia (18%), and surgical-site infections (11%).[13,22] HAIs include VAEs, CLABSIs, CAUTIs, surgical-site infections, and gastrointestinal infections (ie, clostridium (Clostridioides) difficile infection [CDI], formerly known as C difficile).[23,24] In 2018, the Centers for Disease Control and Prevention (CDC)[16] projected that 1 in 31 hospitalized patients had a HAI daily; however, the data for the elderly have not been teased out in this project.

Studies between 2011 and 2023 differ as to which HAIs were responsible for the higher burden of HAIs in individuals aged 65 years and older.[25–35] The foremost microorganisms involved in HAIs among persons aged 65 years and older were E coli, S aureus, Klebsiella species, Pseudomonas aeruginosa, CDI, Acinetobacter species, Enterococcus species, Candida species, Enterobacter species, and Proteus species, of which many of these organisms were MDROs.[35–37]

Recent studies[36,37] have shown that the most common HAIs were respiratory infections followed by UTIs. Pneumonia appeared to be one of the most severe respiratory tract infections among hospital-acquired pneumonia, with VAEs being the most clinically relevant among individuals aged 65 years or older.[30,32] The etiology of UTIs varied between individuals catheterized for less than 30 days and non-catheterized patients and patients with a chronic, indwelling catheter (>30 days).[30,32–35] Sugishita and colleagues[34] found a significant number of individuals with a mean age of 84.8 years who developed a UTI and had a condition (eg, cerebrovascular disorders, neurodegenerative disorders, and diabetes mellitus) that predisposed them to UTI infection.

Skin and soft tissue infections (eg, decubitus ulcers) frequently occur in hospitalized individuals aged 65 years and older, due to intrinsic and extrinsic factors: however, most of these factors are preventable.[34] Intrinsic factors include extended bed confinement due to immobilization, malnutrition, musculoskeletal disorders (eg, bone fractures), and obesity. Extrinsic factors include shear force (eg, sliding down the bed), urine and exudate, and pressure on skin over bony prominences.[30,32,33]

Studies have shown the incidence of CDI is between 4% and 5% higher in individuals a health care facility than healthy individuals (referring only to adults).[37–41] However, there is an 80% mortality rate in individuals aged 65 years or older, due to CDI colitis or toxic megacolon. In addition, there is an increase in length of hospitalization and intra-health care facilities transfers (referring to the movement of an individual within health care facilities) and inter-facility transfers, especially in acute care setting (eg, transfer from the emergency department to an inpatient unit, between 2 or more different units and/or to department for a procedure or diagnostic procedure).[37–41] McHaney-Lindstrom and colleague[41] found that every additional intrahospital transfer, especially in acute care setting, increases the hospitalized individuals' chances of acquiring CDI by 7%.[42–45]

DISCUSSION

In the case of HAIs, efforts for prevention heavily outweigh the complications of HAIs in terms of morbidity, mortality, and associated health care costs. Simple strategies can be adopted by health care facilities to minimize harm to patients by preventing HAIs.[46] The magnitude of the issue of HAIs can be well understood by the importance given to infection prevention by the Joint Commission on Accreditation of Healthcare Organizations (JCAHO).[47] Infection prevention is one of the National Patient Safety Goals (NPSG 07.01.01) and requires health care facilities to improve the quality of health care by instituting measures to prevent infections.

The CDC's National Healthcare Safety Network (NHSN) is a Web-based application utilized nationally by health care facilities to collect data and track health care-associated infections. Data collected are shared with the Centers for Medicare & Medicaid Services (CMS) ensuring compliance with quality measurement reporting requirements, and to local and state health departments upon request. Analysis of collected data is used to foster infection prevention strategies.[48]

The NHSN is in the process of updating national HAI benchmarks (Rebaseline) based on the 2022 data. The method includes data analysis and the creation of risk adjustment models that will be phased in overtime.[49] To track HAIs, NHSN will use a standardized infection ratio (SIR). SIR is a summary measure adjusted based on patient-related (population) and facility factors. SIR is calculated by comparing the actual number of HAI to predicted (baseline data). A SIR of less than 1.0 means that fewer infections than predicted were observed. Conversely, a SIR of greater than 1.0 means that more HAI occurred compared to be predicted. SIR is not calculated when predicted infections are less than 1.0. Using SIR versus infection rate allows for comparison to a national baseline data.[50]

Central Line-Associated Bloodstream Infections

The CDC NHSN defines a central line as "an intravascular catheter that terminates at or close to the heart, or in one of the great vessels, and is used for infusion, withdrawal of blood, or hemodynamic monitoring."[51] Insertion site and type of catheter are not part of the definition. However, type of catheter is reported including permanent central line (tunneled and implanted), temporary (non-tunneled and non-implanted), and umbilical catheters. Specialized catheters (ie, intra-aortic balloon pump, ventricular assist devices, arterial catheters, and certain dialysis accesses) are not considered central lines for reporting. Primary bloodstream infection (BSI) is a laboratory-confirmed infection not linked to an infection at another body site. While a secondary BSI is the result of seeding from a different body location.

Adoption of evidence-based practice guidelines developed by the Society for Healthcare Epidemiology of America in collaboration with several professional organizations Association for Professionals in Infection Control and Epidemiology, Infectious Diseases Society of America, The Joint Commission, and the American Hospital Association and implemented by ACHs has contributed to a 50% drop in CLABSI between 2008 and 2016.[52] According to the most recent, 2022 National and State Healthcare-associated Infections Progress Report, the overall incidence of CLABSI decreased further by 9% between 2021 and 2022. During the same time frame, CLABSI decreased by 21% in intensive care units (ICUs).[53,54]

Recommendations for prevention of CLABSI include judicious usage of central venous catheters (CVCs), utilization of infection control practices to minimize contamination during insertion as well as use of dedicated teams for insertion of catheters, use of antimicrobial, impregnated catheters, antimicrobial lock therapy for long-term CVC usage, and use of antiseptic containing hub/connector cap/port protector to cover all connections.

Catheter-Associated Urinary Tract Infections

A UTI involving any of the organs and structures of the urinary tract that originates from the use of urinary catheters is called a CAUTI. These catheter-associated UTIs are the most common types of the HAIs and account for approximately 75% of UTIs.[54] As per the CDC,[55] 10% to 20% of hospitalized patients receive urinary catheters increasing their risk for CAUTIs. CAUTIs are associated with an increase in length of stay, mortality, morbidity, and health care costs.[56] Advanced age predisposes elderly patients to a higher risk for CAUTIs because of a variety of factors including an increase in dependence on others for self-care, diabetes, malnutrition, high urinary pH, male sex, and prolonged hospitalizations. Prevention strategies for CAUTIs include minimization of urinary catheter usage as well as the duration of usage, use of aseptic insertion techniques, and use of the closed sterile drainage system.[57] There are also specific recommendations for hospitals to develop organizational policies to identify and remove catheters when no longer necessary and create an infrastructure to prevent CAUTIs using best practices. Daily risk of CAUTI remains 3% to 7% with continuous use of catheters. Guidelines regarding education and training of health care professionals in insertion, care, maintenance of urinary catheters, and CAUTI prevention techniques have also been advocated for. A multitude of resources are available to hospitals for CAUTI prevention.[57,58]

Clostridium difficile Infection

CDAD commonly known as C-diff is a known cause of diarrhea associated with antibiotic usage. Approximately 15% to 20% of patients who develop antibiotic-associated diarrhea develop CDI. While use of antibiotics and age are risk factors for CDI, other factors such as gastrointestinal surgery, long stay in the health care settings, underlying illness, and poor immune status also increase the risk for CDI. C Diff spores shed from feces. Contaminated surfaces such as commodes, bathtubs, and rectal thermometers could become a reservoir for the spores that can live on surfaces for a long time. Prevention of C-diff therefore is predominantly dependent on effective management of risk factors through judicious use of antibiotics, thorough handwashing, and effective environmental infection control practices as per CDC recommendations.[59,60]

Ventilator-Associated Events

Approximately, 300,000 critically ill people in the United States require mechanical ventilation each year.[61] While a lifesaving therapy, mechanical ventilation is linked to serious complications including ventilator-associated pneumonia (VAP), pulmonary edema, sepsis, lung injury, and acute respiratory distress syndrome. In 2013, the NHSN implemented new surveillance definition algorithm for VAE. Several changes have been made to the 3 tiered algorithm since inception that includes ventilator-associated condition (VAC), infection-related ventilator-associated complication (IVAC), and possible VAP (PVAP). All adult patients receiving conventional mechanical ventilation or airway pressure release ventilation are included in surveillance data. To be considered a VAE, patients must receive mechanical ventilation on 4 calendar days and demonstrate evidence of infection or inflammation, laboratory evidence of respiratory infection, and/or deterioration in respiratory status after a period of stability or improvement on the ventilator. The detailed VAE algorithm differentiates criteria for VAC, IVAC, and PVAP.

During the early days of the COVID-19 pandemic, patients who tested positive and required mechanical ventilation were at double the risk of VAP compared to ventilate without COVID-19.[9] Fortunately, between 2021 and 2022, VAE decreased 19% in the United States with ICUs reporting an 18% reduction and non-ICUs a 37% decrease, respectively. That said, the SIR for ICUs was 1.200 indicating a higher incidence of VAE than predicted and the need for additional prevention measures.[61,62] Effective handwashing practices by HCWs, head of the bed elevation (30° or higher), minimization of ventilator days, and routine oral care practices to keep the ventilated patient's mouths clean are some effective practices for prevention of VAEs.[63]

Surgical-Site Infection

Approximately, 20% of HAIs are SSI that are associated with increased mortality, longer length of stay, and higher cost of care.[64] The NHSN defines SSI as (1) superficial incisional that only involves skin and subcutaneous tissue; (2) deep incisional that involves fascia and/or muscular; and (3) organ space that includes any body part manipulated during surgery excluding skin incision, fascia, or muscle layers with evidence of infection (purulent drainage, organisms identified by microbiologic testing, or identified by examination [anatomic, histopathologic, or imaging]).

The NHSN monitoring for SSI includes 39 procedures. The 2022 National and State Healthcare-associated Infections Progress Report reports on the 10 Surgical Care Improvement Project procedures.[65] An 8% increase in SSI in patients undergoing hip arthroplasty during 2021 to 2022 was reported. No significant changes related to SSI were found for the other 9 procedures. Risk factors associated with SSI include perioperative characteristics including but not limited to skin preparation, surgical scrub, and antimicrobial prophylaxis; and patient-specific issues including diabetes, obesity, smoking, immunosuppressive therapy, and malnutrition.[66] Controlling the earlier risk factors can be effective in decreasing infections. In addition to effective handwashing practices, skin preparation with chlorhexidine gluconate plus alcohol-based agents, avoidance of razors for skin preparation, maintaining normothermia, decolonization of with intranasal antistaphylococcal agents and antistaphylococcal skin antiseptics for high-risk procedures, perioperative blood glucose control, as well as negative pressure wound therapy have been effective for reducing SSIs.

SUMMARY

Prevention of HAIs is key to decreasing the burden of HAIs. There are several strategies as health care providers we can use to protect HAIs. Considering the higher risk of HAIs in the elderly, extra-attention should be paid to prevent HAIs in the elderly population. These strategies have been discussed and implemented, though the compliance level remains low. Some of these strategies include handwashing for health care professionals and workers, hand hygiene for the patient, early detection of HAIs, isolation, PPE, and antibiotic stewardship.

It has been shown that the most common transmission vectors of HAI pathogens are on the hands of health care workers and handwashing and glove use are the primary prevention strategies health care systems can use to prevent the spread of HAIs to our elderly patients.[67,68] Hand hygiene is the single most important strategy for infection prevention and the JCAHO NPSG underscores the importance of handwashing by requiring health care facilities to prevent infections by ensuring proper handwashing. The most effective approach is to prevent the spread of HAIs from healthcare workers (HCW) hands to the patient through handwashing.[69] Multimodal strategies have been put in place by the World Health Organizations and instrument in health care settings throughout the world. These include alcohol-based hand rub at the point of patient care and/or access to a safe, continuous water supply and soap and towels, training and education of health-care professionals, monitoring of hand hygiene practices and performance feedback, reminders for handwashing, and creation of a hand hygiene safety culture with the participation of HCW and administration.[70] Handwashing campaigns are international and well documented. Patients are encouraged to participate in the handwashing campaign by asking their HCW to wash their hands. Also incorporated into hand hygiene is glove use. Gloves can be misused by providers and studies have shown that when HCW use gloves, their compliance with handwashing with soap and water or an alcohol-based hand rub is low.[3]

Another intervention with low compliance and little discussion is hand hygiene by the patient. Hand hygiene in patients is crucial to prevention of the spread of HAIs as the hands of colonized or infected patients can be contaminated with health care-associated pathogens, which can be transferred to surfaces or the health care providers.[71] It is particularly important to patients ensure that the hands of those colonized or infected with MRSA or CDI participate in hand hygiene because cultures taken from the hands of these patients have been + for their infecting/colonized pathogen.[72,73] Transmission of HAIs and MDRO can occur by simply touching a contaminated surface or object.[74]

In our elderly patients, the authors must be mindful of their limitations when it comes to hand hygiene. Placing towelettes on trays may be difficult for our elderly to open given the changes to their dexterity, or they may have trouble seeing it if they have visual impairment. Hand sanitizers placed on the tray or bedside table can also present challenges, particularly if there are visual impairments or patients have cognitive impairments. Implementation of employee-assisted handwashing and hand sanitizer programs has been shown to increase compliance in handwashing but also a significant decrease in HAI CDI, VRE, and MRSA infection.[75,76]

Not only do we need to ensure that the hands of the patients are clean, but the feet as well. Floors in health care environments have been found to be contaminated with C-Diff spores and MDRO; to prevent this, we should give patients slippers for when they are ambulating in the hallways that can be removed when they get back in bed.[77,78] This will ensure that the spores are not contaminating their nonslip sock and the sheets that patients are laying in for most of their time in the hospital. Contamination of the sheets will also lead to contamination of the patients' hands, clothing, and skin.

Contamination of the patient's skin and clothing can be controlled by changing the patient's clothing every day and allowing the patient to shower over bed bath.[79] Changing patients clothing daily is a routine and easy task; however, showering can prove to be a difficult task for multiple reasons in our elderly. The elderly can have mobility issues, cognitive issues, or visual impairment that may preclude them from showering.

Implementation of these interventions may prove difficult but it is not impossible in the current climate of health care. The shortage of staff will likely make these interventions difficult. It will be a multidiscipline team for the interventions to become successful. Not only would nursing be included, ancillary staff, food services, and even transport would have to participate in these measures for the successful prevention of HAIs in the elderly.[71]

Early detection of HAIs is imperative to stop the spread of these dangerous pathogens. Detecting patients at higher risk to develop HAIs may help prevention or early recognition of the infection. The implementation of bundles can help identify the patients at higher risk for HAIs. Patients who are older than 65 years have increased exposure to antibiotics, immunocompromised, multiple comorbidities, and higher length of stay have higher risk to develop HAIs.[80,81] These patients should be identified early and be monitored for signs and symptoms of HAIs. Should patients exhibit elevated white count, fever, diarrhea, or signs of sepsis; they should be placed in isolation with appropriate personal protective equipment (PPE) until HAIs are ruled out.

Antibiotic stewardship is another effective strategy in the prevention of HAIs. Antibiotic overuse has contributed to the spread of HAIs and the emergence of resistant strains of organisms. Infection prevention teams can help with antibiotic stewardship to decrease the use of broad spectrum and inappropriate antibiotics. Narrowing and optimizing inpatient antibiotic result in increased treatment effectiveness, improve patient safety, and minimize the risk of antibiotic-resistant infections.[82] This is the responsibility of the treating providers. Infection provider capabilities have been limited since the pandemic for a multitude of reasons; therefore, they cannot see every hospitalized patient who is on antibiotics to ensure that the patient is being treated appropriately. Due diligence in providers prescribing antibiotics can help to prevent the emergence of further MDRO in the hospital.

The most common HAIs are MRSA, CDI, and VRE, Acinetobacter, Klebsiella, *E coli*, and Enterobacter. Without appropriate and effective measures put in place to prevent the spread, including diligent hand hygiene, hand hygiene for patients, prevention measures for patients, early recognition of risk factors, and antibiotic stewardship, these HAIs will continue to spread and become drug resistant. In fact, we are now fighting a battle in health care with the MDRO *Candida auris* as a result of the lax prevention measures in health care. *C auris* is a unique challenge because there it is highly transmissible that leads to high number of outbreaks; there are a broad spectrum of clinical manifestations that are associated with a 70% mortality rate; it is environmentally hardy and can remain on dry surfaces for weeks; it is difficult to identify *C auris* by microbiology laboratory; and it has a high rate of MDR and therapeutic failure.[82]

Prompt implementation of multimodal strategies to protect elderly from HAIs may decrease the emergence of new HAIs and hopefully decrease MDROs in circulation.

These measures require systemic process changes, including adequate staffing and education for all involved. These measures will cost health care systems; however, they will prevent senseless deaths and save billions of dollars each year in health care costs. Protecting our vulnerable patients from unnecessary harm while hospitalized should not be an impossible task. Implementation of better hygiene practices for our patients may decrease the spread of pathogens from HCW to patients and patients to HCW. Creating a bundle that would identify patients at high risk for HAIs will allow providers to better screen these patients and allow early detection of HAIs. This would also allow for initiation of isolation and PPE to prevent the spread. Continuing the education and training for all providers on antibiotic stewardship should be a mandatory yearly requirement for those working in high-risk areas, such as inpatient areas and nursing homes. Finally, the authors must continue the hand hygiene campaign in all health care settings. They should accept nothing short of 100% hand hygiene compliance in our health care system. The lack of handwashing in and out of patient care areas is negligent on the part of the HCWs.

CLINICS CARE POINTS

- HAIs pose a burden on the health care system in terms of an increase in morbidity, mortality, length of stay, and health care costs.
- HAIs are preventable.
- Elderly patients are at higher risk of HAIs.
- Prevention strategies require multidisciplinary efforts. Health care providers and health systems must adopt measures to prevent HAIs.
- Handwashing is the single most effective strategy in preventing HAIs.

REFERENCES

1. Worldwide Antimicrobial Resistance National/International Network Group, Collaborators. Ten golden rules for optimal antibiotic use in hospital settings: the warning call to action. World J Emerg Surg 2023;18(1):1–35.
2. Stone PW, Herzig CTA, Agarwal M, et al. Nursing home infection control program characteristics, CMS citations, and implementation of antibiotic stewardship policies: a National Study. Inquiry 2018;55:1–8.
3. Sandbekken IH, Utne I, Hermansen Å, et al. Impact of multimodal interventions targeting behavior change on hand hygiene adherence in nursing homes: an 18-month quasi-experimental study. Am J Infect Control 2024;52(1):29–34.
4. Call E, Call KJ, Oberg C, et al. Healthcare-associated infections and the hospital bed. Adv Skin Wound Care 2023;36(10):1–7.
5. Alanazi Faisal Khalaf, Lapkin S, Molloy L, et al. Healthcare-associated infections in adult intensive care units: a multisource study examining nurses' safety attitudes, quality of care, missed care, and nurse staffing. Intensive Crit Care Nurs 2023;78. N.PAG-N.PAG.
6. Forrester JD, Maggio PM, Tennakoon L. Cost of health care–associated infections in the United States. J Patient Saf 2021. https://doi.org/10.1097/pts.0000000000000845. Publish Ahead of Print.
7. Blot S, Ruppé E, Harbarth S, et al. Healthcare-associated infections in adult intensive care unit patients: changes in epidemiology, diagnosis, prevention and

contributions of new technologies. Intensive Crit Care Nurs 2022;70. https://doi. org/10.1016/j.iccn.2022.103227.

8. Dayanand M, Rao S. Prevention of hospital acquired infections: a practical Guide. Med J Armed Forces India 2004;60(3):312.

9. Cristina ML, Spagnolo AM, Giribone L, et al. Epidemiology and prevention of healthcare-associated infections in geriatric patients: a narrative Review. Int J Environ Res Publ Health 2021;100(10):5333.

10. Jiao P, Jiang Y, Jiao J, et al. The pathogenic characteristics and influencing factors of health care-associated infection in elderly care center under the mode of integration of medical care and elderly care service. Medicine 2021;100(21): e26158.

11. Carestia M, Andreoni M, Buonomo E, et al. A novel, integrated approach for understanding and investigating healthcare associated infections: a risk factors constellation analysis. PLoS One 2023;18(3):e0282019.

12. Zimlichman E, Henderson D, Tamir O, et al. Health care–associated infections. JAMA Intern Med 2013;173(22):2039.

13. Ortman J, Velkoff V and Hogan H, An Aging nation: the older population in the United States population estimates and projections current population reports, Available at: https://www.census.gov/content/dam/Census/library/publications/ 2014/demo/p25-1140.pdf. (Accessed 23 May 2024), 2014.

14. Guzmán-Herrador B, Molina CD, Allam MF, et al. Independent risk factors associated with hospital-acquired pneumonia in an adult ICU: 4-year prospective cohort study in a university reference hospital. J Publ Health 2015;38(2):378–83.

15. Katz MJ, Roghmann MC. Healthcare-associated infections in the elderly. Curr Opin Infect Dis 2016;29(4):388–93.

16. CDC. Healthcare Infection Control Practices Advisory Committee (HICPAC). Healthcare Infection Control Practices Advisory Committee (HICPAC) 2024. Available at: https://www.cdc.gov/hicpac/php/about/index.html. Accessed May 21, 2024.

17. Magill SS, O'Leary E, Janelle SJ, et al. Changes in prevalence of health care–associated infections in U.S. Hospitals. N Engl J Med 2018;379(18):1732–44.

18. Escobar D, Pegues D. Healthcare-associated infections: where we came from and where we are headed. BMJ Qual Saf 2021. https://doi.org/10.1136/bmjqs-2020-012582. bmjqs-2020-012582.

19. Alanazi FK, Lapkin S, Molloy L, et al. Healthcare-associated infections in adult intensive care units: a multisource study examining nurses' safety attitudes, quality of care, missed care, and nurse staffing 2023;78:103480.

20. Association for Professionals in Infection Control and Epidemiology, What are healthcare-associated infections?, Available at: https://apic.org/monthly_alerts/ what-are-healthcare-associated-infections/. (Accessed 20 June 2024).

21. Emori TG, Banerjee SN, Culver DH, et al. Nosocomial infections in elderly patients in the United States. National nosocomial infections surveillance system. Am J Med 1991;91(3b). 289s-93s.

22. Tesini BL, Dumyati G. Health care-associated infections in older adults. Infect Dis Clin 2023;37(1):65–86.

23. Hague M, Sartelli m, McKimm J, et al. Health care-associated infections - an overview. Infect Drug Resist 2018;11:2321–33. Available at: https://pubmed.ncbi.nlm. nih.gov/30532565/.

24. Avci M, Ozgenc O, Coskuner SA, et al. Hospital acquired infections (HAI) in the elderly: comparison with the younger patients. Arch Gerontol Geriatr 2012;54(1): 247–50.

25. Cairns S, Reilly J, Stewart S, et al. The prevalence of health care–associated infection in older people in acute care hospitals. Infect Control Hosp Epidemiol 2011;32(8):763–7.

26. Thompson N, Stone N, Brown C, et al. Prevalence and epidemiology of healthcare-associated infections (HAI) in US nursing homes (NH), 2017. Infect Control Hosp Epidemiol 2020;41(S1):s45–6.

27. Nelson RE, Hyun D, Jezek A, et al. Mortality, length of stay, and healthcare costs associated with multidrug-resistant bacterial infections among elderly hospitalized patients in the United States. Clin Infect Dis 2022;74(6):1070–80.

28. Cristina ML, Spagnolo AM, Giribone L, et al. Epidemiology and prevention of healthcare-associated infections in geriatric patients: a narrative review. Int J Environ Res Publ Health 2021;18(10):5333.

29. Abbasi SH, Aftab RA, Mei Lai PS, et al. Prevalence, microbial etiology and risk factors associated with healthcare associated infections among end stage renal disease patients on renal replacement therapy. J Pharm Pract 2022. https://doi.org/10.1177/08971900221094269. 089719002210942.

30. Alrebish SA, Yusufoglu HS, Alotibi RF, et al. Epidemiology of healthcare-associated infections and adherence to the HAI prevention strategies. Healthcare 2022; 11(1):63.

31. Schattner A. The spectrum of hospital-associated harm in the elderly. Eur J Intern Med 2023;115:29–34.

32. Liang S, Wang Y, Wang WL, et al. Characteristics of hospitalized elderly patients with CKD: a comparison between elderly and non-elderly CKD based on a multicenter cross-sectional study. Int Urol Nephrol 2023;56(2):625–33.

33. Stewart S, Robertson C, Pan J, et al. Epidemiology of healthcare-associated infection reported from a hospital-wide incidence study: considerations for infection prevention and control planning. J Hosp Infect 2021;114:10–22.

34. Esme M, Topeli A, Yavuz BB, et al. Infections in the elderly critically-ill patients. Front Med 2019;6(118).

35. Cillóniz C, Rodríguez-Hurtado D, Rodríguez-Hurtado D, et al. Characteristics and management of community-acquired pneumonia in the era of global aging. Med Sci 2018;6(2):35.

36. van Someren Gréve F, Juffermans NP, Bos LDJ, et al. Respiratory viruses in invasively ventilated critically ill patients-a prospective multicenter observational study. Crit Care Med 2018;46(1):29–36.

37. Jump RLP, Crnich CJ, Mody L, et al. Infectious diseases in older adults of long-term care facilities: update on approach to diagnosis and management. J Am Geriatr Soc 2018;66(4):789–803.

38. Martin-Loeches I, J Schultz M, Vincent JL, et al. Increased incidence of co-infection in critically ill patients with influenza. Intensive Care Med 2016;43(1):48–58.

39. Sugishita K, Saito T, Iwamoto T. Risk factors for nursing- and healthcare-associated urinary tract infection. Geriatr Gerontol Int 2018;18(8):1183–8.

40. Yoshikawa TT, Norman DC. Geriatric infectious diseases: current concepts on diagnosis and management. J Am Geriatr Soc 2017;65(3):631–41.

41. Lessa FC, Mu Y, Bamberg WM, et al. Burden of Clostridium difficile infection in the United States. N Engl J Med 2015;372(9):825–34.

42. Asempa T, Nicolau D. Clostridium difficile infection in the elderly: an update on management. Clin Interv Aging 2017;12:1799–809.

43. Bristol AA, Schneider CE, Lin SY, et al. A systematic review of clinical outcomes associated with intrahospital transitions. J Healthc Qual 2019;42(4):1.

44. McHaney-Lindstrom M, Hebert C, Flaherty J, et al. Analysis of intra-hospital transfers and hospital-onset Clostridium difficile infection. J Hosp Infect 2019;102(2): 168–9.

45. Bush K, Barbosa H, Farooq S, et al. Predicting hospital-onset *Clostridium difficile* using patient mobility data: a network approach. Infect Control Hosp Epidemiol 2019;40(12):1380–6.

46. An ounce of prevention is worth a pound of cure. Merriam-Webster.com dictionary, Merriam-Webster. Available at: https://www.merriam-webster.com/dictionary/anounceofpreventionisworthapoundofcure. Accessed September 13, 2024.

47. The Joint Commission. National patient safety goals for hospitals. Available at: https://www.jointcommission.org/-/media/tjc/documents/standards/national-patient-safety-goals/2024/npsg_chapter_hap_jan2024.pdf. (Accessed 14 September 2024), 2024.

48. Centers for Disease Control and Prevention, NHSN's stated purposes, Available at: https://www.cdc.gov/nhsn/about-nhsn/technology.html. (Accessed 14 September 2024), 2023.

49. Centers for Disease Control and Prevention, Charting the course: 2022 HAI rebaseline, Available at: https://www.cdc.gov/nhsn/pdfs/rebaseline/22-Rebaseline-FAQs-Final-Version.pdf. (Accessed 14 September 2024), 2024.

50. Centers for Disease Control and Prevention, The NHSN standardized infection ratio (SIR), Available at: https://www.cdc.gov/nhsn/pdfs/ps-analysis-resources/nhsn-sir-guide.pdf. (Accessed 14 September 2024), 2024.

51. National Healthcare Safety Network, Bloodstream infection event (central line-associated bloodstream infection and non-central line associated bloodstream infection), Available at: https://www.cdc.gov/nhsn/pdfs/pscmanual/4psc_clabs current.pdf. (Accessed 14 September 2024), 2024.

52. Beville ASM, Heipel D, Vanhoozer G, et al. Reducing central line associated bloodstream infections (CLABSIs) by reducing central line days. Curr Infect Dis Rep 2021;23:23.

53. Buetti Niccolò, Marschall J, Drees M, et al. Strategies to prevent central line-associated bloodstream infections in acute-care hospitals: 2022 Update. Infect Control Hosp Epidemiol 2022;43(5):553–69. https://doi.org/10.1017/ice.2022.87.

54. Buetti N, Marschall J, Drees M, et al. Strategies to prevent central line-associated bloodstream infections in acute-care hospitals: 2022 Update. Infect Control Hosp Epidemiol 2022;43(5):553–69.

55. Centers for Disease Control and Prevention. Clinical safety for healthcare providers. Available at: https://www.cdc.gov/uti/hcp/clinical-safety/index.html. Accessed September 9, 2024.

56. Chant C, Smith OM, Marshall JC, et al. Relationship of catheter- associated urinary tract infection to mortality and length of stay in critically ill patients: a systematic review and meta-analysis of observational studies. Crit Care Med 2011;39: 1167–73.

57. Patel PK, Advani SD, Kofman AD, et al. Strategies to prevent catheter-associated urinary tract infections in acute-care hospitals: 2022 Update. Infect Control Hosp Epidemiol 2023;44(8):1209–31.

58. Association for Professionals in Infection Control and Epidemiology. Catheter-associated urinary tract infection. Available at: https://apic.org/resources/topic-specific-infection-prevention/catheter-associated-urinary-tract-infection/. Accessed September 2, 2024.

59. Centers for Disease Control and Prevention. Clinical overview of Clostridioides difficile infection. Available at: https://www.cdc.gov/c-diff/hcp/clinical-overview/. Accessed September 2, 2024.

60. Centers for Disease Control and Prevention. Guideline for the prevention of healthcare-associated infections: environmental infection control. Available at: https://www.cdc.gov/infection-control/media/pdfs/Guideline-Environmental-H.pdf. Accessed September 4, 2024.

61. Centers for Disease Control and Prevention. 2022 National and state healthcare-associated infections progress report. 2023. Available at: https://www.cdc.gov/healthcare-associated-infections/media/pdfs/2022-Progress-Report-Executive-Summary-H.pdf. Accessed September 2, 2024.

62. National Healthcare Safety Network. Ventilator-associated event (VAE). 2024. Available at: https://www.cdc.gov/nhsn/pdfs/pscmanual/10-vae_final.pdf. Accessed August 20, 2024.

63. Centers for Disease Control and Prevention. Ventilator-associated pneumonia: about. Available at: https://www.cdc.gov/ventilator-associated-pneumonia/about/index.html. Accessed September 2, 2024.

64. Klompas Michael. Ventilator-associated pneumonia, ventilator-associated events, and nosocomial respiratory viral infections on the leeside of the pandemic. Respir Care 2024;69(7):854. *Gale Academic OneFile*. . Accessed September 9, 2024.

65. National Healthcare Safety Network. Surgical site infection event (SSI). 2024. Available at: https://www.cdc.gov/nhsn/pdfs/pscmanual/9pscssicurrent.pdf. Accessed September 9, 2024.

66. Calderwood Michael S, Anderson DJ, Bratzler DW, et al. Strategies to prevent surgical site infections in acute-care hospitals: 2022 Update. Infect Control Hosp Epidemiol 2023;44(5):695–720.

67. Seidelman JL, Mantyh CR, Anderson DJ. Surgical site infection prevention: a review. JAMA 2023;329(3):244–52.

68. Facciolà A, Pellicanò GF, Visalli G, et al. The role of the hospital environment in the healthcare-associated infections: a general review of the literature. Eur Rev Med Pharmacol Sci 2019;23(3):1266–78.

69. Bolcato V, Robustelli della Cuna FS, Fassina G, et al. Preventing healthcare-associated infections: hand disinfection monitoring using an automated system in an Italian neurological hospital. Healthcare 2023;11(23):NA. Gale Academic OneFile. Accessed 16 Sept. 2024.

70. WHO Guidelines on hand hygiene in healthcare. World Health Organisation. Available at: www.who.int/publications/i/item/9789241597906. Accessed April 21, 2020.

71. Donskey Curtis J. Empowering patients to prevent healthcare-associated infections. Am J Infect Control 2023;51(11):A107–13.

72. Bobulsky GS, Al-Nassir WN, Riggs MM, et al. Clostridium difficile skin contamination in patients with C. difficile–associated disease. Clin Infect Dis 2008;46(3):447–50. Print.

73. Chang S, Sethi AK, Eckstein BC, et al. Skin and environmental contamination with methicillin-resistant staphylococcus aureus among carriers identified clinically versus through active surveillance. Clin Infect Dis 2009;48(10):1423–8.

74. Jury A, Guerrero DM, Burant CJ, et al. Effectiveness of routine patient bathing to decrease the burden of spores on the skin of the patient with CDI. Infect Control Hosp Epidemiol 2010;32:181–4.

75. Gagné D, Bédard G, Maziade PJ. Systematic patients' hand disinfection: impact on meticillin-resistant Staphylococcus aureus infection rates in a community hospital. J Hosp Infect 2010;75(45):269–72.
76. Pokryuka M, et al. Can improving patient hand hygiene impact CDI events in an Academic Medical Center. Am J Infect Control 2017;45:954–64.
77. Torres-Teran MM, Alhmidi H, Koganti S, et al. Dissemination of methicillin-resistant Staphylococcus aureus and bacteriophage MS2 from floors in long-term care facility resident rooms. Am J Infect Control 2023;51(6):714–7.
78. Haq MF, Alhmidi H, Redmond SN, et al. A Randomized Control Trial to determine whether wearing slippers decreases bacteriophage MS2 from patient surfaces to hospital rooms. Infect Control Hosp Epidemiol 2023;44(4):670–3.
79. Otter JA, Vickery K, Walker JT, et al. Surface-attached cells, biofilms and biocide susepibilty: implications for hospital cleaning and disinfecting. J Hosp Infect 2015;89(1):16–27.
80. Ayada G, Atamna A, Babich T, et al. Community versus health care-associated Clostridioides difficile infection: a comparison between clinical characteristics and outcomes in hospitalized patients. Am J Infect Control 2023;51(12):1339–43.
81. Abbasi SH, Aftab RA, Mei Lai PS, et al. Prevalence, microbial etiology and risk factors associated with healthcare associated infections among end stage renal disease patients on renal replacement therapy. J Pharm Pract 2023;36(5):1142–55.
82. O'Connor M, McNamara C, Doody O. Healthcare workers' experiences of caring for patients colonized with carbapenemase-producing Enterobacterales (CPE) in an acute hospital setting - a scoping review. J Hosp Infect 2023;131:181–9.

Management of Neutropenic Fever in Persons with Cancer

Susan Doyle-Lindrud, DNP, APN

KEYWORDS

- G-CSF • Neutrophils • Cancer • Chemotherapy • Immunosuppression
- Granulocytopenia • Prophylaxis • Risk stratification

KEY POINTS

- Neutropenic fever is a medical emergency requiring prompt evaluation and treatment with broad spectrum antibiotics to prevent life-threatening sepsis.
- Febrile neutropenia is a significant cause of morbidity and mortality in patients with cancer.
- A risk assessment tool, such as the Multinational Association of Supportive Care in Cancer and/or Clinical Index of Stable Febrile Neutropenia can be utilized to guide the decision as to whether a patient with neutropenic fever requires hospital admission and intravenous antibiotics or can be managed as an outpatient.
- Preventive measures for neutropenic fever include primary prophylaxis with granulocyte colony-stimulating factor (G-CSF) in appropriate patients, such as those with prolonged neutropenia.

BACKGROUND

Neutrophils, or polymorphonuclear granulocytes (PMNs), are the most common type of white blood cell and are produced in bone marrow. Neutrophils are the first line of defense as part of the innate immune system, and act by killing invading organisms such as bacteria and fungi. When neutrophils encounter signs of an infection, they respond by phagocytosis, intracellular degradation, release of granules, and formation of neutrophil extracellular traps. Neutrophils are also mediators of inflammation.[1] When the neutrophil count is low, the immune system is compromised and there is an increased risk of recurrent infections.

Neutropenia is defined as an absolute neutrophil count (ANC) below 1.5×10^9/L (1500/mm³). Neutropenia can be further classified as mild (ANC $1.0–1.5 \times 10^9$/L), moderate ($0.5–1.0 \times 10^9$/L), severe ($0.2–0.5 \times 10^9$/L), and very severe (<0.2×10^9/L) (**Table 1**).[2,3] Febrile neutropenia is defined by the Infectious Disease Society of America, American Society of Clinical Oncology (ASCO), and the National Comprehensive

Columbia University School of Nursing, 560 West 168th Street, New York, NY 10032, USA
E-mail address: Smd9@cumc.columbia.edu

Nurs Clin N Am 60 (2025) 479–489
https://doi.org/10.1016/j.cnur.2024.09.004
0029-6465/25/© 2024 Elsevier Inc. All rights are reserved, including those for text and data mining, AI training, and similar technologies.

Table 1
Absolute neutrophil count grading criteria

Grade	Absolute Neutrophil Count Range (Cells/mm³)	Severity
Normal	> 1500	-
1	1000–1500	Mild
2	500–999	Moderate
3	< 500–1000	Severe
4	< 500	Life-threatening

Adapted from Justiz Vaillant AA, Rout P, Reynolds SB, et al. Neutropenia. [Updated 2024 Jun 7]. In: StatPearls [Internet]. Treasure Island (FL): StatPearls Publishing; 2025 Jan-. Available from: https://www.ncbi.nlm.nih.gov/books/NBK507702/. Disclosure: Preeti Rout declares no relevant financial relationships with ineligible companies. Disclosure: Samuel Reynolds declares no relevant financial relationships with ineligible companies. Disclosure: Patrick Zito declares no relevant financial relationships with ineligible companies. 2024.

Cancer Network (NCCN) as a single oral temperature $\geq$38.3°C (101.0° F), or a sustained temperature $\geq$ 38.0°C (100.4°F) for 1 hour, and an ANC less than 0.5 × 10⁹/L or an ANC that is expected to decrease to less than 0.5 × 10⁹/L within 48 hours.[4] When the cause of neutropenia is related to chemotherapy treatment for a cancer patient, a dose reduction and/or a delay in subsequent treatment cycle is a potential consequence. Due to patient safety concerns, febrile neutropenia leads to emergency department evaluations and hospitalizations. An infection in a neutropenic patient can increase morbidity and mortality and without a prompt evaluation, can lead to sepsis, septic shock syndrome, and death.[5]

RISK FACTORS FOR NEUTROPENIA

Neutropenia is a serious complication of cancer chemotherapy. Many standard chemotherapy regimens for solid tumors result in 6 to 8 days of neutropenia with 5% to 30% of patients developing febrile neutropenia.[6] Patients undergoing hematopoietic stem cell transplantation with a conditioning regimen or receiving chemotherapy for a hematologic malignancy have a longer duration of neutropenia, sometimes lasting 14 days or more, with more than 80% developing neutropenic fever.[7] Chemotherapy regimens are classified as being high risk (>20%), intermediate risk (10%–20%), or low risk (<10%) of developing febrile neutropenia. Other factors that increase risk of developing febrile neutropenia include $\geq$ 65 years of age, having advanced disease, having had a prior febrile neutropenia episode, poor performance status, renal and liver dysfunction, low body surface area, and specific genetic polymorphisms.[8,9] Other causes of neutropenia include radiation therapy if given to areas of red bone marrow, such as the pelvis and sternum; hematologic tumors such as lymphomas, leukemias, and multiple myeloma; solid tumors that infiltrate the bone marrow; or other disorders that affect the bone marrow such as myelodysplastic syndromes. Infections can cause neutropenia, such as coronavirus disease 2019, Epstein Barr virus, human immunodeficiency virus, and hepatitis. Nutritional deficiencies can also cause neutropenia, such as low vitamin B12, copper, or folate. There is also chronic idiopathic neutropenia, which is a neutropenia without a clear cause.[10]

INITIAL EVALUATION

When a patient presents to an emergency department with a fever and they have had chemotherapy within the past 6 weeks, it should be assumed that they may have a bacterial infection. The vital signs, including temperature, should be obtained and the fever should be documented. Lab tests should be drawn, including a complete blood count with leukocyte differential count, hemoglobin and platelet count, serum electrolytes, serum creatinine, blood urea nitrogen, and liver function tests including total bilirubin, alkaline phosphatase, aspartate transaminase and alanine transaminase. At least 2 sets of blood cultures should be drawn from different sites, including a peripheral location as well as from a central venous catheter if the patient has one. In addition, cultures from other sites such as urine, stool, and/or respiratory tract should be obtained as indicated. Patients should have a comprehensive evaluation that includes a complete history and physical examination, with a systematic approach that focuses on identifying a potential infection. The physical examination should include an evaluation of the skin, lungs, sinus, mouth, abdomen, perirectal area, neurologic system, and catheter site(s), as these are potential sources of infection. Important considerations include medical comorbidities, type of chemotherapy regimen and timing of most recent treatment, ill contacts, social history, travel history, and recent antibiotic therapy or prophylaxis. For patients presenting with symptoms and/or signs of a respiratory infection, chest imaging and a sputum culture should be obtained, and respiratory viral testing should be considered during influenza season.[6,11]

Patients with febrile neutropenia require prompt evaluation and initiation of antibiotics. The Infectious Disease Society of America (IDSA), the National Comprehensive Cancer Network (NCCN), and the ASCO recommend a risk assessment utilizing a scoring system, such as the Multinational Association of Supportive Care in Cancer (MASCC) or the Clinical Index of Stable Febrile Neutropenia (CISNE). These risk assessment tools identify low-risk patients that might be good candidates for outpatient management.[12]

RISK ASSESSMENT

The MASCC risk index is an internationally validated scoring system that identifies the low-risk patients that can potentially be treated with oral antibiotics as an outpatient. The factors considered to determine the score include burden of illness (symptoms), hypotension, whether the patient has active chronic obstructive pulmonary disease (COPD), the type of cancer, and age of the patient (**Table 2**). Higher scores indicate lower risk, with a maximum of 26 points. Patients with an MASCC score $\geq$ 21 are

Table 2 Multinational Association of Supportive Care in Cancer risk index	
Characteristic	**Score**
Burden of illness: no or mild symptoms	5
No hypotension (systolic blood pressure > 90 mm Hg)	5
No chronic obstructive pulmonary disease	4
Solid tumor or no previous fungal infection	4
No dehydration	3
Burden of illness: moderate symptoms	3
Outpatient status	3
Age <60 y	2

Adapted from Taplitz RA, Kennedy EB, Bow EJ, et al. Outpatient Management of Fever and Neutropenia in Adults Treated for Malignancy: American Society of Clinical Oncology and Infectious Diseases Society of America Clinical Practice Guideline Update. Journal of Clinical Oncology. 2018;36(14):1443-1453.

considered to be low risk for complications. If a patient is low risk and the neutropenic length is anticipated to be less than 7 days, the patient can tolerate and absorb oral medication and is available for close follow-up from the health care provider, then outpatient antibiotics can be considered. If the patient does not meet these criteria, or the patient has documented drug-resistant infection or gastrointestinal intolerance of oral antibiotics, then inpatient intravenous (IV) antibiotics are indicated. Patients with a score less than 21 are considered high risk for serious complications of febrile neutropenia, such as death, intensive care unit admission, and hypotension. If the MASCC score is high risk, then inpatient IV antibiotics are indicated.[4]

The second risk stratification score that can be used to identify the low-risk febrile neutropenic patient is the (CISNE). This tool is used for adults 18 years and older in the outpatient setting who have a solid tumor and a fever of 100.4°F (38° C) for over 1 hour in duration and neutropenia defined by 500 cells/mm^3 or 1000 cells/mm^3 with an expected drop to 500 cells/mm.^{3} The tool looks at Eastern Cooperative Oncology Group (ECOG) performance status, stress-induced hyperglycemia, COPD, cardiovascular disease history, National Cancer Institute (NCI) mucositis grade ≥ 2, and monocytes count, each category being assigned a numeric value (**Table 3**). A 0-point score on the tool is considered low risk of complications and the health care provider could consider outpatient management of this patient. Intermediate risk is a score of 1 to 2, and the health care provider should use clinical judgment regarding admission. A high-risk score is ≥ 3 and this patient should be admitted to the hospital.[13] A systematic review and meta-analysis of the MASCC and CISNE scores for predicting serious complications has been conducted. The pooled sensitivity and specificity for MASCC less than 21 were 55.6% (95% CI: 46.2%–64.5%) and 86% (95% CI:81.3%–89.7%), respectively. The pooled sensitivity and specificity for CISNE ≥ 1 were 96.7% (95% CI: 93.6%–98.3%) and 22.2% (95% CI: 15.6%–30.4%), respectively. The conclusion of the study was that the CISNE score might be more useful in an acute setting due to the higher sensitivity.[12]

Table 3	
Clinical index of stable febrile neutropenia	
Characteristic	**Points**
Eastern Cooperative Oncology Group (ECOG) Performance Status	
≥ 2	2
History of Chronic Obstructive Pulmonary Disease	
Yes (Emphysema, chronic bronchitis, decreased forced expiratory volumes, or need for oxygen therapy, corticosteroids, or bronchodilators)	1
Cardiovascular Disease	
Yes (Cor pulmonale, heart failure, cardiomyopathy, hypertensive heart disease, valvular heart disease, or other structural malformations)	1
Mucositis Grade ≥ 2	
Yes (Presence of patchy ulcerations or pseudomembranes; or moderate pain with modified diet indicated)	1
Monocyte Count	
$< 0.2 \times 10^9$/L	1
Stress-Induced Hyperglycemia	2

Adapted from Taplitz RA, Kennedy EB, Bow EJ, et al. Outpatient Management of Fever and Neutropenia in Adults Treated for Malignancy: American Society of Clinical Oncology and Infectious Diseases Society of America Clinical Practice Guideline Update. Journal of Clinical Oncology. 2018;36(14):1443-1453.

MANAGEMENT

When a patient with neutropenic fever arrives at the emergency department, the first dose of antibiotic therapy should be given within 1 hour. If the degree of risk for the patient is not yet known or is known to be high, then the patient should receive IV therapy with an antipseudomonal β-lactam drug, such as cefepime or piperacillin-tazobactam.[4,14] Vancomycin should be considered if there are concerns for a catheter-related infection, soft tissue infection, or hemodynamic instability. Modifications should be considered to the initial antibiotic therapy regimen if the patient is found to have an antibiotic-resistant organism, including methicillin-resistant *Staphylococcus aureus*, in which one would initiate vancomycin, linezolid, or daptomycin or a vancomycin-resistant *Enterococcus*, in which one would consider treating with linezolid or daptomycin.[4,14] For extended-spectrum β-lactamase-producing gram-negative bacteria, one should consider carbapenem. For a *Klebsiella pneumoniae carbapenemase* infection, one should consider polymyxin-colistin or tigecycline or a new β-lactam with activity against gram-negative resistant organisms.[11]

If the patient has a penicillin allergy, a cephalosporin can be considered, but if the patient has a history of a hypersensitivity reaction such as bronchospasm, this patient should instead be treated with ciprofloxacin plus clindamycin or aztreonam plus vancomycin.[6,11]

In high risk patients with hematologic malignancies who have an anticipated neutropenia of greater than 7 days, a fungal infection should be considered and may require additional imaging depending on the symptoms.[6] Discontinuation of antibiotics can be considered if a patient has a fever of unknown origin and is hemodynamically stable and afebrile for 48 hours, regardless of ANC count and expected duration of neutropenia.[15]

If the risk is low, the patient can receive oral or IV antibiotics. It is recommended that the first dose of antibiotics be given in the clinic or emergency department and the patient should be observed over a minimum of 4-hour duration before discharge. If a patient's fever responds to initial antibiotic treatment and the patient remains stable, they may be eligible to continue treatment as an outpatient. Other considerations in deciding whether a patient can be treated as an outpatient include whether the patient lives ≤ 30 miles from the clinic or hospital; the oncologist agrees with outpatient management; the patient has a family member available as caregiver; the patient has access to a telephone and transportation; the patient has a history of compliance with treatment regimens; and the patient agrees to frequent telephone communication with the health care provider for follow-up monitoring.[11]

Outpatient management of neutropenic fever includes the oral antibiotic regimen of ciprofloxacin plus amoxicillin clavulanate. Alternative options include levofloxacin or ciprofloxacin single agent or ciprofloxacin plus clindamycin.[11] The length of the antibiotic regimen is dictated by the organism and the site. The antibiotic regimen should continue until the ANC is greater than 500 cells/mm^3.

If the patient's fever has not gone away after 2 to 3 days of starting the antibiotic, the regimen may need to be adjusted, and the patient should be evaluated for readmission to the hospital. Reasons for readmission include new signs of infection, inability to take oral medications, blood cultures becoming positive, or microbiologic testing identifies an organism not sensitive to current regimen.[11]

RISK REDUCTION STRATEGIES

Patients on chemotherapy, radiation, and/or a biologic therapy that is myelosuppressive, require education due to the risk of neutropenia. It is important for patients to understand the timing that neutropenia will likely develop based on the treatment given. The patient should be counseled on how to monitor for signs and symptoms of infection, such as fever, cough, chills, diarrhea, dysuria, erythema, or pain. The patient should be provided information on who to call if they develop symptoms or fever after treatment and should be provided with a backup plan if this contact is not available, such as going to the emergency room with a notecard stating the treatment the patient is on, date of last treatment, and the oncologist contact information.[16]

Neutropenic patients are at risk of food-borne illness due to organisms such as *Escherichia coli*, *Klebsiella*, *Pseudomonas,* and *Proteus*. Because these organisms can be found in fresh fruits and vegetables, over the past 2 decades, health care providers have been recommending a low-bacterial diet, otherwise known as a cooked diet or neutropenic diet. The belief has been that by avoiding fresh fruits and vegetables, patients with neutropenia would have a lower risk of developing a food-borne infection. Sonbol and colleagues (2019), conducted a systematic review and meta-analysis of 6 studies (5 randomized controlled trials and 1 observational study), looking at the effectiveness of neutropenic diets in decreasing infection and mortality in neutropenic cancer patients. The study found no statistically significant difference in infection rates (relative risk [RR] 1.16; 95% CI 0.94–1.42) or mortality (RR 1.08; 95% CI 0.78–1.50) in patients with chemotherapy-induced neutropenia on a neutropenic diet as compared to a regular diet. The American Cancer Society, ASCO, and the IDSA guidelines now recommend patients instead be counseled on safe food handling practices as recommended by the US Food and Drug Administration. This includes washing hands before preparing a meal, rinsing fresh fruit and vegetables under warm running water, scrub or brush produce to remove excess dirt, use separate cutting boards for meat and produce, and avoid non pasteurized dairy products and undercooked meat and eggs.[17] During a hospitalization, good hand and oral hygiene is important for preventing hospital-acquired infections. Good skin care should include daily showers or baths and these patients should have thorough skin examinations, including assessment of catheter sites and the perineum. Rectal thermometers, suppositories, and enemas should be avoided.[4]

The gut microbiome has been found to be a potential source of bacterial infections that can cause neutropenic fever, but now studies are also revealing that the gut microbiome may be a contributor to neutropenic fever not caused by an infection in patients after chemotherapy. A study by Shwabkey, Z. et al (2022), evaluated 119 patients undergoing a hematopoietic stem cell transplant, all who developed neutropenia. Of the total 119 patients, 56 of these patients remained afebrile and 63 developed a fever, with 7 developing a bloodstream infection. All patients had a microbiome analysis at the onset of neutropenia and it was found that patients who developed a fever had an increase of the mucin-degrading bacteria *Akkermansia muciniphila* as compared to those patients that did not develop fever (54% vs 32%, respectively; $P = .02$).[18]

The investigators then looked at preclinical mouse models via in vivo and in vitro analysis, examining how radiation, chemotherapy, antibiotics, and calorie restriction affect the gut microbiome. They found that chemotherapy, radiation, and calorie restriction increased *A muciniphila* and thinned the colonic mucus layer. Treatments for cancer often decrease appetite which may increase this mucus-degrading activity, possibly increasing the risk for neutropenic fever. Focusing on nutritional support when counseling patients who are undergoing chemotherapy might be a beneficial approach to reducing toxicities of cancer treatment.[18]

Mobile technologies are showing promise in improving patient monitoring while neutropenic cancer patients are at home. A case series by Nessle, and colleagues

(2022), describes 3 pediatric cancer patients who were found to have a fever at home, detected 5 to 12 hours prior to the thermometer findings of fever due to a high-frequency temperature monitoring wearable device. The earlier finding of fever in these patients led to an earlier clinical evaluation. Two of the three children with fever had a bloodstream infection. Because of the wearable device, an earlier intervention and initiation of antibiotics was possible.[19]

Remote medical care via synchronous and asynchronous technology has been on the rise over the past decade and both patient and provider have become more comfortable with this approach, especially during the coronavirus disease 2019 pandemic. Wearable devices will continue to be an increasingly important tool that can be utilized by health care providers for the purpose of remote monitoring of oncology patients' vital signs, electrocardiogram, activity levels, etc. while the patient remains at home, with a goal of identifying problems earlier.[20]

ANTIMICROBIAL PROPHYLAXIS

ASCO and IDSA guidelines recommend antimicrobial prophylaxis with antibacterial and/or antifungals for patients considered high-risk for febrile neutropenia or have an anticipated length of neutropenia (ANC <100 cells/mm^3) of greater than 7 days or other factors that increase risk for complications or mortality. ASCO and IDSA recommend oral fluoroquinolones as an antibacterial and an oral triazole for antifungal prophylaxis. If a chemotherapy regimen has an increased risk (>3.5%) for pneumonia from *Pneumocystis jirovecii*, then trimethoprim-sulfamethoxazole is recommended. If a patient is herpes simplex virus seropositive undergoing allogeneic hematopoietic stem cell transplant, then a nucleoside analog such as acyclovir is recommended.[21] Antimicrobial prophylaxis is not recommended in low-risk patients.[15]

HEMATOPOIETIC GROWTH FACTORS

To reduce the risk of infection, recombinant human granulocyte colony stimulating factor (G-CSF) has been used for many years to decrease the length of neutropenia in patients on chemotherapy. G-CSF stimulates the production, maturation, and activation of neutrophils in the bone marrow. Filgrastim was the first G-CSF approved for febrile neutropenia prevention in 1991.[22] Since this time, many biosimilars, which are biologically similar products, have been developed for use, which has decreased cost burden for these medications, including filgrastim-sndz and tbo-filgrastim. The original filgrastim dosing regimen had been found to be very inconvenient for patients due to requirements to come to the clinic or hospital once daily for several days after their chemotherapy treatment for the injection. Pharmaceutical research has since led to the development of a long-acting drug that requires dosing only once per cycle. This long-acting medication was developed through the addition of polyethylene glycol (PEG) to colony stimulating factor (PEGylation), which due to the PEG component, decreased its clearance from the body until the neutrophils recovered.[23] More recently, due to the development of a wearable delivery method for pegfilgrastim, such as Onpro, which is an injector placed on the skin of a cancer patient after receiving chemotherapy, patients no longer need to return to the clinic for this injection. The injector automatically delivers pegfilgrastim approximately 27 hours after application. The patient is then given instructions on how to remove and dispose of the injector themselves at home based on health care provider instructions.[24]

Filgrastim or tbo-filgrastim, is dosed at 5 mcg/kg, given subcutaneously to the patient daily, until the post nadir ANC has recovered. The injection should begin 24 hours after chemotherapy or up to 3 to 4 days after completion of the chemotherapy cycle.

Pegfilgrastim is dosed at 6 mg and should be given subcutaneously 24 hours after the chemotherapy dose, although it can be given up to 3 to 4 days after chemotherapy. It should be given at least 12 days prior to the next cycle of chemotherapy.[25]

The NCCN guideline recommends G-CSF be given as primary prophylaxis with the first cycle of chemotherapy when a regimen has a 20% risk or higher of neutropenia. When a patient is on a chemotherapy regimen with an intermediate risk (10%–20%) of neutropenia, then primary prophylaxis should be considered for those who have 1 or more risk factors. Some examples of risk factors include prior chemotherapy or radiation, persistent neutropenia, bone marrow infiltration of tumor, and age greater than 65 years. Patients do not typically need primary prophylaxis with G-CSF if they are on a low-risk regimen. Secondary G-CSF prophylaxis occurs when a patient develops an episode of febrile neutropenia after a subsequent cycle of chemotherapy. These patients become high risk for future febrile neutropenia episodes and the decision is often made to initiate G-CSF with ongoing cycles at that time.[25]

NOVEL NEW AGENTS

There are novel medications that are now available for the prevention and treatment of chemotherapy-induced neutropenia and neutropenic fever. Trilaciclib is a small molecule inhibitor of cyclin-dependent kinase 4/6. This drug is Food and Drug Administration approved to decrease the incidence of chemotherapy-induced myelosuppression in patients on platinum/etoposide or topotecan-based chemotherapy for extensive stage small cell lung cancer. It works by temporarily arresting the hematopoietic stem cells and progenitor cells in the G1 phase of the cell cycle, which protects these cells from damage from chemotherapy. Trilaciclib is given as an IV infusion at a recommended dose of 240mg/m^2 over 30 minutes and is initiated within 4 hours of the start of chemotherapy on each day treatment is given.[5]

Efbemalenograstim alfa-vuxw is a long-acting colony stimulating factor that works similarly to G-CSF, by acting on hematopoietic cells to stimulate growth of neutrophils. It helps by boosting the immune function of cancer patients and is indicated in adult patients with non-myeloid cancers receiving chemotherapy who have a significant risk of febrile neutropenia. It is given as a 20 mg subcutaneously injection once per chemotherapy cycle, approximately 24 hours after treatment.[5,26]

Eflapegrastim-xnst is a long-acting recombinant human granulocyte growth factor that binds to the G-CSF receptors on myeloid progenitor cells and increases the number of mature circulating neutrophils, leading to a decrease in the incidence of infection. It is indicated for adult patients with non-myeloid cancers receiving chemotherapy associated with a significant risk of febrile neutropenia. Eflapegrastim-xnst is given as a 13.2 mg subcutaneous injection 24 hours after chemotherapy.[5]

Plinabulin is an investigational, first in class non-GCSF selective immunomodulating microtubule binding agent. Plinabulin has an early onset of action in chemotherapy-induced neutropenia by boosting the number of hematopoietic stem cells/progenitor cells and by triggering the release of an immune defense protein, guanine nucleotide exchange factor H1 (GEF-H1), which may lead to an anticancer benefit. Plinabulin is currently in 2 global multi-center clinical trials evaluating the prevention of chemotherapy-induced neutropenia in non-myeloid cancers.[27]

SUMMARY

Febrile neutropenia is a serious complication of myelosuppressive treatment, and fever might be the only sign of infection that an oncology patient presents with. Management of these patients includes a prompt comprehensive evaluation by a health care provider and initiation of antibiotics within 1 hour of presentation to the clinic or emergency department. Important considerations include the type of chemotherapy, comorbidities, stage of cancer, prior therapies, and the current ANC. A risk assessment utilizing a scoring system, such as the MASCC or CISNE, should be obtained to help identify the low-risk patients that might be good candidates for outpatient management. Empiric antibiotics should be given promptly to patients with neutropenic fever to help reduce morbidity and mortality rates and considerations for the need for hematopoietic growth factors for future treatments should be considered.

CLINICS CARE POINTS

- Obtain blood cultures from each lumen of the central venous catheter and peripherally before starting antibiotics.
- Use risk stratification tools like MASCC or CISNE to help guide inpatient versus outpatient management, but exercise clinical judgment.
- For high-risk patients, admit for IV antibiotics with antipseudomonal coverage (eg, cefepime, piperacillin-tazobactam).
- Low-risk patients may be candidates for outpatient oral antibiotics (eg, fluoroquinolone ± amoxicillin-clavulanate), but require close monitoring.
- Continue antibiotic treatment until ANC is greater than 500 cells/mm^3 and patient is afebrile for at least 48 hours.

REFERENCES

1. Holland SM, Gallin JI. Disorders of granulocytes and monocytes. In: Loscalzo J, Fauci A, Kasper D, et al, editors. Harrison's principles of internal medicine. 21e. New York, NY: McGraw-Hill Education; 2022.
2. Justiz Vaillant AA, Rout P, Reynolds SB, et al. Neutropenia. In: StatPearls. Treasure Island (FL): with ineligible companies; 2024. Disclosure: Preeti Rout declares no relevant financial relationships with ineligible companies. Disclosure: Samuel Reynolds declares no relevant financial relationships with ineligible companies. Disclosure: Patrick Zito declares no relevant financial relationships with ineligible companies.
3. Boccia R, Glaspy J, Crawford J, et al. Chemotherapy-induced neutropenia and febrile neutropenia in the US: a beast of burden that needs to be tamed? Oncol 2022;27(8):625–36.
4. Freifeld AG, Bow EJ, Sepkowitz KA, et al. Clinical practice guideline for the use of antimicrobial agents in neutropenic patients with cancer: 2010 update by the infectious diseases society of America. Clin Infect Dis 2011;52(4):e56–93.
5. Blayney DW, Schwartzberg L. Chemotherapy-induced neutropenia and emerging agents for prevention and treatment: a review. Cancer Treat Rev 2022;109:102427.
6. Zimmer AJ, Freifeld AG. Optimal management of neutropenic fever in patients with cancer. J Oncol Pract 2019;15(1):19–24.
7. Stohs EJ, Abbas A, Freifeld A. Approach to febrile neutropenia in patients undergoing treatments for hematologic malignancies. Transpl Infect Dis 2024;e14236.
8. Averin A, Silvia A, Lamerato L, et al. Risk of chemotherapy-induced febrile neutropenia in patients with metastatic cancer not receiving granulocyte colony-stimulating factor prophylaxis in US clinical practice. Support Care Cancer 2021; 29(4):2179–86.

9. Lyman GH, Abella E, Pettengell R. Risk factors for febrile neutropenia among patients with cancer receiving chemotherapy: a systematic review. Crit Rev Oncol Hematol 2014;90(3):190–9.

10. Frater JL. How I investigate neutropenia. Int J Lab Hematol 2020;42(Suppl 1): 121–32.

11. Taplitz RA, Kennedy EB, Bow EJ, et al. Outpatient management of fever and neutropenia in adults treated for malignancy: American society of clinical oncology and infectious diseases society of America clinical practice guideline update. J Clin Oncol 2018;36(14):1443–53.

12. Zheng B, Toarta C, Cheng W, et al. Accuracy of the Multinational Association of Supportive Care in Cancer (MASCC) and Clinical Index of Stable Febrile Neutropenia (CISNE) scores for predicting serious complications in adult patients with febrile neutropenia: a systematic review and meta-analysis. Crit Rev Oncol Hematol 2020;149:102922.

13. Coyne CJ, Le V, Brennan JJ, et al. Application of the MASCC and CISNE risk-stratification scores to identify low-risk febrile neutropenic patients in the emergency department. Ann Emerg Med 2017;69(6):755–64.

14. Contejean A, Maillard A, Canoui E, et al. Advances in antibacterial treatment of adults with high-risk febrile neutropenia. J Antimicrob Chemother 2023;78(9): 2109–20.

15. Dickter J, Logan C, Taplitz R. Neutropenia and antibiotics: when, what, how and why? Curr Opin Infect Dis 2023;36(4):218–27.

16. Foley AM, Hoffman M. CE: febrile neutropenia in the chemotherapy patient. Am J Nurs 2023;123(5):36–42.

17. Sonbol MB, Jain T, Firwana B, et al. Neutropenic diets to prevent cancer infections: updated systematic review and meta-analysis. BMJ Support Palliat Care 2019;9(4):425–33.

18. Schwabkey ZI, Wiesnoski DH, Chang CC, et al. Diet-derived metabolites and mucus link the gut microbiome to fever after cytotoxic cancer treatment. Sci Transl Med 2022;14(671):eabo3445.

19. Nessle CN, Flora C, Sandford E, et al. High-frequency temperature monitoring at home using a wearable device: a case series of early fever detection and antibiotic administration for febrile neutropenia with bacteremia. Pediatr Blood Cancer 2022;69(9):e29835.

20. Closs K, Verket M, Muller-Wieland D, et al. Application of wearables for remote monitoring of oncology patients: a scoping review. Digit Health 2024;10. 2055207 6241233998.

21. Taplitz RA, Kennedy EB, Bow EJ, et al. Antimicrobial prophylaxis for adult patients with cancer-related immunosuppression: ASCO and IDSA clinical practice guideline update. J Clin Oncol 2018;36(30):3043–54.

22. Aghedo BO, Gupta V. Filgrastim. In: StatPearls. Treasure Island (FL): ineligible companies; 2024. Disclosure: Vikas Gupta declares no relevant financial relationships with ineligible companies.

23. De Oliveira Brandao C, Lewis S, Sandschafer D, et al. Two decades of pegfilgrastim: what have we learned? Where do we go from here? Curr Med Res Opin 2023; 39(5):707–18.

24. Parker SD, King N, Jacobs TF. Pegfilgrastim. In: StatPearls. Treasure Island (FL): ineligible companies; 2024. Disclosure: Nafisa King declares no relevant financial relationships with ineligible companies. Disclosure: Tibb Jacobs declares no relevant financial relationships with ineligible companies.

25. Griffiths EA, Roy V, Alwan L, et al. NCCN guidelines(R) insights: hematopoietic growth factors, version 1.2022. J Natl Compr Cancer Netw 2022;20(5):436–42.
26. Crawford J, Oswalt C. The impact of new and emerging agents on outcomes for febrile neutropenia: addressing clinical gaps. Curr Opin Oncol 2023;35(4):241–7.
27. BeyondSpring. Plinabulin. 2024. Available at: https://beyondspringpharma.com/pipeline/plinabulin/. Accessed June 8, 2024.

Overview of the Epidemiology, Diagnosis, and Clinical Care Considerations for People Living with and at Risk for Tuberculosis in the United States

Alanna Bergman, PhD, AGNP-BC, RN[a],*, Tania Thomas, MD, MPH[b]

KEYWORDS

- Tuberculosis • TB • TPT • Isolation

KEY POINTS

- Tuberculosis (TB) remains a significant threat to public health in the United States disproportionately burdening marginalized and vulnerable communities.
- There are 4 TB centers of excellence funded through the Centers for Disease Control that offer resources and support to health care workers who would like additional TB education, resources, and clinical consultation.
- Tuberculin skin test and interferon-gamma release assay are 2 effective and accessible tests for effective TB screening; each has benefits and should be selected based on the client's situation.
- There are 3 recommended regimens for TB prophylaxis that should be offered to people with identified TB infection that has not progressed to TB disease.
- The Infectious Disease Society of America has published new guidance for isolation to reduce community TB transmission; using new evidence and a person-centered lens, these guidelines prioritize least restrictive means to reduce transmission while mitigating the psychological and social impacts of isolation.

[a] School of Nursing, University of Virginia, 202 Jeanette Lancaster Way, PO Box 800782, Charlottesville, VA 22903, USA; [b] Division of Infectious Diseases and International Health, University of Virginia School of Medicine, University of Virginia, PO Box 801340, Charlottesville, VA 22908-1340, USA
* Corresponding author.
E-mail address: dhm8ax@virginia.edu

Nurs Clin N Am 60 (2025) 491–506
https://doi.org/10.1016/j.cnur.2024.10.004
0029-6465/25/© 2024 Elsevier Inc. All rights are reserved, including those for text and data mining, AI training, and similar technologies.
nursing.theclinics.com

INTRODUCTION AND EPIDEMIOLOGY OF TUBERCULOSIS IN THE UNITED STATES

Despite recent advances in pharmacotherapy and health care infrastructure, tuberculosis (TB) remains a leading infectious killer globally.[1] This is unsurprising given that more than 10 million people are diagnosed with TB every year.[1] The United States has a relatively low incidence of TB.[1] However, TB stills occur in the United States; the year 2023 saw an 8% increase in TB cases compared with pre-coronavirus disease 2019 (COVID-19) pandemic levels in 2019.[2] In 2023, New York City alone experienced a 28% increase in TB cases[3] (536 diagnostically confirmed cases), the highest rate in more than a decade.[3] This increase followed a markedly low number of diagnoses recorded in 2020, likely due to reduced case finding resulting from the COVID-19 pandemic. In 2022 and 2023, 2 separate outbreaks of TB in the United States were tied to bone grafts containing live cells from a deceased donor with clinical symptoms of TB.[4] This oversight led to 10 known deaths and required treatment of more than 100 individuals.[4] These outbreaks are unfortunate and preventable.

Most adult TB cases in the United States occur among people born in other countries.[2] Among those born in the United States, TB cases are generally reflective of larger health disparities along racial and ethnic lines.[2] Although they make up a minority of the population, Black and Latino persons make up 60% of TB cases in the United States.[2] TB incidence is highest among indigenous Americans (American Indians and Alaska Natives) and Hawaiian and Pacific Islanders.[5] Other disparities in TB are driven by socioeconomic status. People who are unhoused and/or living in shelters are more likely to develop TB disease.[6] Similar research indicates that in the United States, people who are unemployed, unhoused, or use substances are more likely to die of TB disease.[7]

The Center for Disease Control and Prevention (CDC) has stratified US cities and states into 3 categories: high-incidence, moderate-incidence, and low-incidence TB areas. The classification is based on cases per 100,000 persons with a national average of 2.4 cases per 100,000 and most cases occur in Alaska, California, Maryland, New York, and Texas.[8]

The World Health Organization has a lofty goal toward TB elimination by the year 2035[9] that will require additional resources to ensure timely diagnosis of TB disease, linkage to care and treatment, as well as robust case investigations to locate and screen individuals with exposure to TB and initiate preventative treatment to prevent progression where appropriate. To halt the ongoing spread of TB in the community, clinicians and public health officials must have a strong working knowledge of TB to be able to screen, identify, refer, and treat clients who present for care.

STRUCTURE OF TUBERCULOSIS RESOURCES IN THE UNITED STATES

Fortunately, in the United States, there are a variety of TB training and educational services available to nurses and health care providers ranging from paper resources and infographics, to online classes, to in-person training, and consultation services. These resources are funded by the CDC's TB education and consultative services and are available through 4 TB centers of excellence. These centers are based on geographic location (**Fig. 1**) and include the Curry International Tuberculosis Center that serves the Western United States, the Mayo Clinic Center of Tuberculosis for the mid-west and Texas, the Global TB Institute at Rutgers University servicing the Northeastern United States, and the Southeastern National TB Center that supports the South East and Illinois. Nurses and other health care providers who require training, consultation, and support in management of complex TB disease are encouraged to contact the centers of excellence (1–800–4TB-INFO [1–800–482–4636]) to be connected to a training program or medical provider with expertise in your area of clinical need.

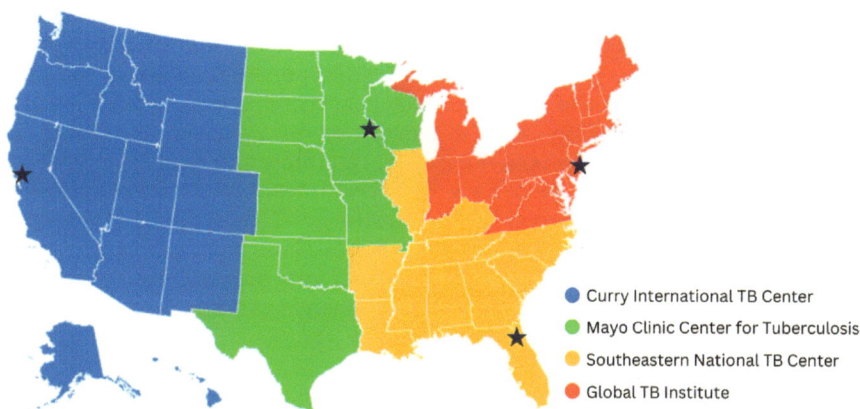

Fig. 1. Areas of coverage for the tuberculosis centers of excellence. Note: Map lines delineate study areas and do not necessarily depict accepted national boundaries. Stars indicate approximate location of each TB center of excellence.

WHAT CAUSES TUBERCULOSIS AND HOW IS IT SPREAD?

TB is caused by *Mycobacterium tuberculosis* (*Mtb*), a slow-growing aerobic bacterium identified by Robert Koch in 1882.[10] *Mtb* belongs to a genus of bacteria called acid-fast bacillus that also include *Mycobacterium leprae*, the causative agent in Hansen's disease (leprosy), and *Mycobacterium avium complex* that is pervasive in the human environment and has been isolated in environmental dust, dirt, and water.[11] TB can affect any organ or tissue but most commonly affects the lungs causing the characteristic cough and hemoptysis that pulmonary TB is known for. TB is spread from person to person through airborne particles called droplet nuclei.[12,13] Traditionally, *Mtb* particles were thought to be spread through the air primarily via cough, as coughing expels large volumes of droplet nuclei. However, other activities such as singing and talking also contribute to droplet expulsion[14] and recent evidence indicates that tidal breathing may account for a large percentage of TB transmissions.[15,16] Once an individual is exposed to *Mtb* and the bacillus proceeds into the lower respiratory tract, alveolar macrophages initiate a complex process in which the body attempts to rid itself of *Mtb*. In some cases, the macrophages, cytokines, and dendritic cells of the immune system are successful and the host expels the *Mtb* effectively clearing the infection, but in other cases, the immune system instead attempts to isolate, control, and wall off the bacillus to prevent further dissemination within the host.[17] This process can culminate in the TB granuloma, a "chronic inflammatory lesion,"[18] which may or may not be successful in preventing progression to TB disease.

Exposure

Exposure to TB is necessary but not sufficient to cause infection or disease. Development of TB disease is dependent on 4 factors: (1) host susceptibility, (2) infectiousness of the person expelling TB particulates, (3) factors in the environment, and (4) exposure.[19]

Susceptibility refers to the clinical and genetic factors that increase or decrease an individual's likelihood of developing clinical TB after exposure. Some individual predisposing factors, such as human immunodeficiency virus (HIV), diabetes, and age less than 5 years, are well documented in the literature.[1] These individual factors limit the host's ability to contain the *Mtb,* increasing the risk of disease progression. There is also a clear link between genetics and TB susceptibility but the specific pathways through which this occurs remain opaque.[20,21] While genetic factors may remain unclear for some time, clinicians should consider host immunocompetence when evaluating TB risk. Susceptibility also includes several variables associated with socioeconomic status, for example, nutrition that can more than double the risk of progression from TB infection to disease.[22] A large recent randomized control trial demonstrated that nutrition support is an effective anti-TB intervention[23] highlighting the role that undernutrition plays in TB susceptibility. Given high rates of food insecurity in North America, and the cost-effectiveness of food access programs, undernutrition should be considered a high priority for preventing TB progression.

Infectiousness

Infectiousness often refers to the bacillary burden of the person with TB disease. When considering infectiousness, first consider the location of TB disease. Individuals with localized extrapulmonary TB such as liver, bone, or brain TB without lung involvement cannot transmit aerosolized droplets and should be considered noninfectious.[24] For those with pulmonary TB, bacillary burden can be evaluated through several factors that we will describe in depth (1) presence or absence of cavitary disease, (2) smear positivity, and (3) initiation of anti-TB treatment.[25] Cavities are believed to form when the center of a TB granuloma becomes filled with air, leaving an oxygen rich compartment where bacteria can replicate efficiently.[26] Due to limited vascularity of necrotic areas surrounding the cavity, there is poor penetration of both immune cells and antitubercular drugs, and therefore, bacterial growth continues unchecked.[26] These areas of high-bacillary accumulation lead to higher rates of mortality for the person with TB disease, and higher relative risk of transmission to others.[25] Until recently, smear positivity was one of the most widely accepted indicators of host infectiousness.[27] Some evidence supports that individuals with positive smears who have not yet initiated anti-TB therapy are potentially more infectious than those with negative smears.[25] However, there is newer evidence indicating that smear status may not be a clinically significant predictor of transmissibility and is particularly unreliable in the presence of anti-TB treatment.[28] This evidence suggests that transmission risk warrants a much larger view of risk factors, beyond sputum status. Newer guidelines call for the use of a variety of individual data points to evaluate infectious risk.[24] Initiation of anti-TB treatment is the single most important factor in evaluating infectiousness. Ample evidence displays the rapid bactericidal effect of combination therapy on culture positivity,[27,29] with some studies indicating a 50% decrease in culturable *Mtb* in fewer than 2 days of treatment.[30] Similarly, in studies evaluating human transmission to animals, individuals started on effective anti-TB treatment do not readily transmit to guinea pigs despite great vulnerability to *Mtb*.[31] All of these factors indicate that rapid initiation of effective anti-TB therapy interrupts *Mtb* transmission, negating the role of sputum positivity as a marker of infectivity after treatment initiation.[24]

Environment

The environment is an undeniable factor in TB transmission. Overcrowding and poor ventilation in indoor spaces are 2 of the most significant environmental factors increasing transmission risk in *Mtb*.[12,32] Settings that cluster large groups of individuals indoors such as schools and public transportation (ie, buses, trains) are important sites of transmission.[33] Other institutions such as homeless shelters and prisons are well known for their propensity for TB transmission not only due to overcrowding and poor ventilation but also because these institutions often bring together people with increased susceptibility to TB creating an environment ripe for transmission.[34-36] While households that contain a person living with TB present a risk to other household contacts, several studies in high-burden areas indicate that most transmission occurs outside of the home, in the community.[33,37,38]

Exposure

There are a variety of factors that influence exposure risk in TB transmission. When evaluating exposure, the clinician must consider the frequency, duration, and proximity of exposure. In essence, how often and how closely was an individual in contact with someone with TB? Increased frequency and duration of contact with *Mtb* increase the individual's risk for infection. Undiagnosed individuals generally have long periods of exposure to other household contacts that underpins the focus and policies of contact tracing.

WHAT IS THE DIFFERENCE BETWEEN TUBERCULOSIS INFECTION AND TUBERCULOSIS DISEASE?

Traditionally, clinicians categorized people into TB infection (previously called latent TB) and TB disease (previously called active disease). TB infection indicates exposure and immunologic evidence of infection with *Mtb* without clinical symptoms or radiologic/ bacteriologic evidence of disease. People with TB infection are not able to transmit *Mtb* and most remain asymptomatic containing the infection through sustained immune response.[24] A small proportion of people (4%–6%) go on to develop TB disease that can occur imminently after infection, or more often, disease progresses years after initial infection.[39] TB disease generally produces symptoms (fever, cough, night sweats, anorexia, weight loss, etc., though symptoms differ based on location and extent of disease dissemination) and radiologic evidence of disease on chest radiograph. People with clinical disease do transmit *Mtb* via cough and respiratory aerosolization. In contrast to the historically binary schema, recent science has indicated a third and important category of people, those with subclinical TB.[40] Drain and colleagues[41] define subclinical TB as "disease due to viable *Mtb* bacteria that does not cause clinical TB-related symptoms but causes other abnormalities that can be detected using existing radiologic or microbiologic assays." In line with this most recent evidence, we now acknowledge that TB may occur on a continuum ranging from exposure through disease.[42,43] Engaging people in care requires not only active case finding for those with symptoms, but robust contact investigation to assess close contacts of people with TB disease, screening high-risk individuals, and initiation of appropriate treatment or prophylaxis. A recent modeling study estimated that nearly 3% of the US population is infected with *Mtb*, equivalent to more than 8 million people[44] reasserting the importance of screening and treating TB infection.

HOW TO IDENTIFY TUBERCULOSIS EXPOSURE?

There are 2 well-validated tests approved for TB screening. The tuberculin skin test (TST) uses an intradermal injection of 0.1 mL of purified protein derivative into the skin of the forearm to evaluate local immune response to *Mtb*.[39] TSTs were developed in 1944 and quickly became the international standard for screening for then termed latent TB. TSTs are easily stored in a clinic refrigerator and can be administered by nursing staff and medical assistants. However, correct placement requires training and expertise to produce a wheal (an elevation in skin created by the injected tuberculin derivative); if no wheal appears, this may indicate incorrect administration and invalidate the test.[39] After placement, the client must return to the clinic within 48 to

72 hours for interpretation.[39] Because tests are also read by clinical staff, there is some degree of subjectivity as they measure the presence and degree of induration or swelling. Erythema is not indicative of a positive test and should not be measured or considered in test interpretation.[39] TSTs are classified and interpreted according to baseline risk for TB disease with higher tolerated thresholds for lower risk groups. More than 5 mm of induration is considered positive for the highest risk groups including people with HIV, contacts to TB, and people who are immunosuppressed due to a chronic condition or medication. More than 10 mm of induration is considered positive for people of moderate risk, including people born in TB-endemic countries, people who engage in hazardous alcohol or drug use, young children, people with chronic medical conditions placing them at risk for TB (diabetes, severe kidney disease, malignancy, etc.), inhabitants of high-risk living situations such as nursing homes, correctional facilities and housing shelters, and people with occupational exposure to TB. Finally, induration of 15 mm or more is considered positive for the lowest risk group of people with no known TB risk factors (**Fig. 2**). If the TST test is invalidated due to errors in administration or failure to return for interpretation, the test may be repeated. According to the CDC, there is no risk of repeated TST placements.[45] TSTs require very little equipment aside from a 27 gauge tuberculin syringe that are relatively inexpensive and often readily available in clinic spaces.

Interferon-γ release assays (IGRAs) measure cellular immune response of T cells to *Mtb* antigen. Two IGRAs are commercially available in the United States for screening for TB infection, QuantiFERON Plus, and T-SPOT.TB. While both TST and IGRA tests can accurately identify TB infection, there is evidence that IGRAs demonstrate greater accuracy in predicting incident TB disease.[46] Unlike the TST test that reacts to the presence of other mycobacterial species, IGRAs are specific to *Mtb*. IGRAs must be processed in a laboratory and thus do not require a return clinic visit. The laboratory reports a qualitative result (positive; negative) corresponding to the quantitative cell-mediated response[47]; this process greatly reduces subjectivity in interpretation. While the Infectious Disease Society of America prefers the IGRA over TST for testing for TB infection in those with low-to-moderate risk of progression to TB disease, or those likely to be infected with *Mtb*, they also acknowledge the utility of the TST as a valid and reliable test and endorse TST when cost or burden would prohibit the use of IGRAs.[39] Similarly, the American Academy of Pediatrics recognizes that neither test is perfectly sensitive for the diagnosis of TB infection; however, recent studies have

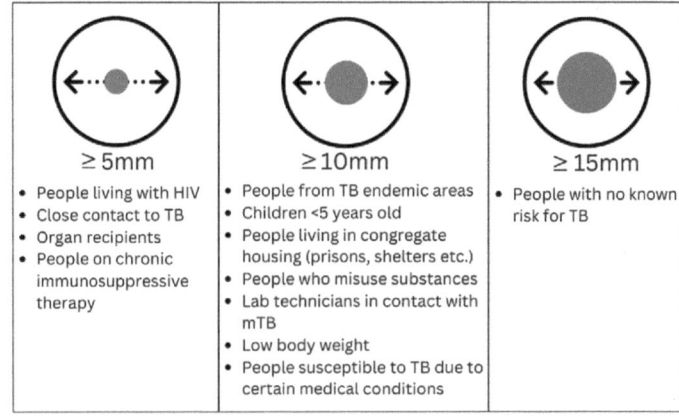

Fig. 2. Measurement for TST interpretation.

demonstrated that IGRAs are an acceptable alternative to TSTs in children of any age, including those less than 2 years.[48,49]

Both TST and IGRAs can be used for screening for TB infection; however, neither test can differentiate between TB infection and disease. Once a client develops a positive response to either test, additional history, screening, and/or testing is necessary to rule out TB disease. It is essential to rule out TB disease prior to initiating treatment of TB infection (latent TB) or risk development of resistance further complicating treatment (see **Fig. 3** for a graphic depicting the pros and cons of each screening test).

WHAT ARE THE TREATMENT RECOMMENDATIONS FOR TUBERCULOSIS INFECTION WITHOUT DISEASE (LATENT TUBERCULOSIS)?

The National Tuberculosis Coalition of America, in conjunction with the CDC, endorses several treatment options for latent TB infection chosen for their efficacy, tolerability, and limited duration.[50] Treatment choice should consider pill burden, comorbid conditions, polypharmacy and drug–drug interactions, and patient preference based on individual psychosocial needs. First-line regimens include (1) 3 months of weekly isoniazid plus rifapentine (3HP), (2) 4 months of daily rifampin (4R), and (3) 3 months of daily isoniazid plus rifampin (3HR; **Fig. 4**).[50] These 3 options are preferred over 2 alternative regimens of 6 or 9 months of daily isoniazid. While daily isoniazid is effective and was the standard treatment regimen for many years, prolonged exposure to isoniazid is associated with higher rates of hepatotoxicity and other adverse effects that may lead to discontinuation, or dwindling adherence due to the long-extended nature of treatment.[50] Some evidence suggests that the vast majority of people initiated on TB preventive therapy will never complete their prophylaxis. Therefore, treatment selection should be made in conjunction with the patient, prioritizing shorter treatment duration when possible to promote adherence.

WHAT ARE THE TREATMENT RECOMMENDATIONS FOR LABORATORY-CONFIRMED TUBERCULOSIS DISEASE?

Since 2016, the standard treatment of culture-positive pulmonary TB was 6 months of daily treatment including 2 months of isoniazid, rifampin, pyrazinamide and ethambutol (HRZE), followed immediately by 4 months of isoniazid and rifampin.[51]

In 2022, the CDC published "Interim guidance: the use of a 4 month rifapentine-moxifloxacin regimen for treatment of drug-susceptible pulmonary tuberculosis." The guidance and adoption of this new regimen as a recommended treatment option[52] were established following publication of data indicating non-inferiority of the isoniazid,

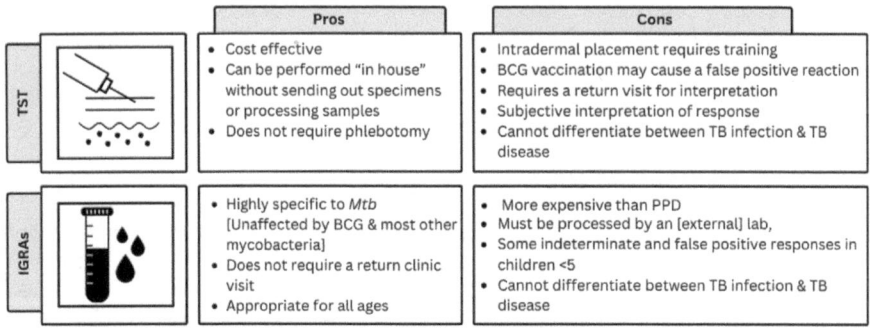

Fig. 3. Pros and cons of TST versus IGRA.

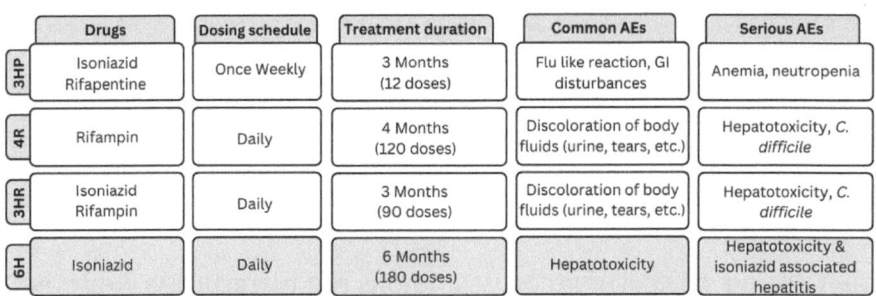

Fig. 4. CDC recommended regimens for tuberculosis preventive therapy.

rifapentine, moxifloxacin and pyrazinamide (HPMZ) regimen compared to the previous standard 6 month HRZE regimen.[53] This new regimen shortens treatment duration of drug-sensitive pulmonary TB by 2 months and includes 8 weeks of daily isoniazid, rifapentine, moxifloxacin, and pyrazinamide, followed by 9 weeks of daily isoniazid, rifapentine, and moxifloxacin. Though a 4 month regimen, the total treatment length is 17 weeks.[52] The intensive phase has a clinically significant pill burden compared to the standard HRZE regimen. Including prophylactic pyridoxine, the HPMZ regimen comprises 15 tablets taken once daily then reduced to 11 tablets after the initial 8 weeks. The HPMZ regimen is only appropriate for adults and adolescents at least at the age of 12 years, weighing more than 40 kg with laboratory-confirmed pulmonary TB.[52] This regimen is not appropriate for people who are pregnant or breastfeeding, those with confirmed or high suspicion for extrapulmonary TB, or those with known resistance to any of the medications in the treatment regimen, including the fluoroquinolone class.[52]

The rifamycin drug class, which includes rifabutin, rifampin, and rifapentine, is essential to the treatment and prophylaxis of Mtb.[39,51,52] It is important to note that medications in this drug class are moderate-to-strong inducers of the CYP3A4 pathway and accelerate the metabolism of some drugs.[54] This enhanced metabolism can result in lower concentrations of some coadministered drugs resulting in underexposure and can lead to toxic exposure of some metabolites.[54] It is best practice to utilize interaction-checking technology through your institution before initiation of new medications during or immediately following TB treatment or prophylaxis.

In primary care and infectious disease settings in the United States, people with TB disease are managed by public health departments who handle the specifics of dosing, treatment duration, and management of adverse effects. However, most initial TB diagnostics are conducted outside of the public health system[39] and clinicians should be familiar with basic principles diagnosis and treatment and should be aware of common drug–drug interactions and adverse effects. For more specific information regarding the treatment of culture-confirmed pulmonary TB, please refer to "The Official American Thoracic Society/Centers for Disease Control and Prevention/Infectious Diseases Society of America Clinical Practice Guidelines: Treatment of Drug-susceptible Tuberculosis"[51] and the CDC's Interim guidance document.[52]

DRUG RESISTANCE IN TUBERCULOSIS

Drug resistance is a major concern in the treatment of TB.[1] Treatment interruption/discontinuation, insufficient treatment, and treatment failure all contribute to TB mortality and development of drug-resistant TB.[55] In the global community, rifampicin and isoniazid susceptibility is under threat but drug-resistant TB is currently limited in the United States. In 2022, 8.4% of all TB cases diagnosed in the United States were resistant to isoniazid, and 1.4% of cases were confirmed multi-drug resistant.[56] In order to maintain high sensitivity to our recommended regimens, HRZE and HPMZ, we must help clients to achieve high levels of treatment adherence particularly during the intensive phase of treatment when chances of acquired drug resistance are highest.[57] To do this, many districts employ directly observed therapy (DOT), either in person or virtually to verify adherence,[58] but use of DOT should remain individualized based on client specific needs.

ISOLATION GUIDELINES

In June 2024, the TB Coalition of America, in conjunction with the Infectious Disease Society of America, issued new guidelines for respiratory isolation of people with TB in the community. Isolation and quarantine have always been a cornerstone of public health strategies to reduce TB transmission. However, prevailing policies did not

---

Box 1
Summary of recommendations for respiratory isolation from the National Tuberculosis Coalition of America and Infectious Disease Society of America

Recommendation 1—Goals of respiratory isolation and restrictions
- 1.1 TB respiratory isolation and restriction should consider the potential benefits and harms for the community at large, and for people with TB.

Recommendation 2—Defining respiratory isolation and restrictions
- 2.1 Respiratory isolation and individual restrictions should be conceived as a spectrum (from no restriction, to extensive restrictions such as quarantine, or restriction of visitors) that are tailored for individuals with TB, and their biologic and social conditions (see guideline for additional details and guiding framework).

Recommendation 3—Determining infectiousness and transmission risk
- 3.1 Prior to initiation of effective treatment, people who have higher respiratory burden of *Mtb* (ie, sputum smear and/or nucleic acid amplification test [NAAT]) positivity, cavitation on chest imaging) can be considered relatively more infectious than those with lower bacillary burden considering individual circumstances.
- 3.2 People with TB on less than 5 days of effective therapy should be considered relatively more infectious than those on longer durations of effective treatment.
- 3.3 People with TB on effective treatment for 5 days or more should be considered noninfectious or with a low likelihood of infectiousness, regardless of sputum status.
- 3.4 When considering overall risk of TB transmission to others, clinicians should consider all factors contributing to transmission: host infectiousness, exposure, environment, and contact susceptibility.

Recommendation 4—Determining whether community-based respiratory isolation is indicated
- 4.1 Respiratory isolation is not recommended for people without infectious forms of TB (ie, localized extrapulmonary TB).
- 4.2 People on effective treatment and with low likelihood of infectiousness should not have restriction in *most* circumstances.
- 4.3 Respiratory restriction and/or isolation may be considered for people who have higher risk of infectious transmission.

Recommendation 5—Determining level of respiratory isolation and restriction
- 5.1 A moderate range of restriction should be considered appropriate for people with TB in most circumstances.
- 5.2 Choice of respiratory restriction and duration of restriction/isolation should be reassessed at a minimum of once weekly and should be modified based on evolving circumstances.
- 5.3 When respiratory restrictions are implemented, clinicians should provide support to mitigate harm to the person with TB.

See full guidelines for additional detail about each recommendation and the evidence used to support individual recommendations.

Table 1
Practical suggestions for reducing barriers to treatment

Barrier to Care	Potential Solution
Individual barriers to care	
Financial barriers • Food insecurity • Housing instability • Cost of care • Lack of transportation • Fear of work disruptions	• Referral to clinic-based social workers or social service for help applying for food and housing assistance • Refer clients to co-pay programs or 340B programs for reduced pharmacy costs • Provision of travel vouchers (may be eligible from state and local governments based on income and/or age) • Provide employers with documentation of health needs (with client's consent) and assist with medical leave paperwork if appropriate.
Knowledge and literacy barriers • Low TB self-efficacy • Low health literacy • Low perceived seriousness of TB infection/disease • Fear of side effects/toxicity	• Individualized health education, tailored to literacy and educational level (ie, providing video or visual information in lieu of text) • Comprehensive TB education • Include client's preferences in regimen selection if possible to minimize fears of toxicity and polypharmacy.
Forgetfulness • Forgetting or missing doses	• Assisting client with alarms, reminder devices, and adherence applications • Reinforcing significance of missed doses and why adherence to treatment is prioritized
Intrapersonal Barriers	
Perceived lack of support • Family/social support • Medical support	• If available and appropriate, utilize peer navigators to increase social support and care navigation • With the client's consent, provide education to family and friends to increase TB knowledge, reduce fears of transmission, and increase social support • Prioritize provider continuity to build rapport and trust • Offer adherence, and social support visits

Social stigma	• Reaffirm individual personhood throughout treatment by:
	  ○ Using person-centered language
	  ○ Including the client in care decisions when possible
	  ○ Acknowledging the unique nuances of individual health and care needs
	• Decrease social isolation by utilizing the least restrictive isolation methods while minimizing transmission risk
	• Reassess the need for quarantine and isolation frequently (at least weekly)
	• Counsel family members and household contacts about TB to increase knowledge and reduce misinformation

Organizational Barriers	
Clinic location	• Establish mobile clinics if possible • Offer telehealth visits for education and follow-up • Consider nurse visits to the client's home for education, follow-up, and TST interpretation

(continued on next page)

Table 1 (*continued*)	
Barrier to Care	**Potential Solution**
Provider availability	• Employ task-shared models with nurses and community health workers to increase health care worker availability • Offer evening and weekend clinics to accommodate work and caregiving schedules
Isolation and quarantine	• Apply new National TB Coalition of America guidelines for respiratory isolation using least restrictive measures to reduce transmission of TB while considering the mental and emotional well-being of the person with TB
DOT	• For TB treatment, use of creative directly observed therapy when appropriate (ie, electronic or video directly observed therapy, DOT at a client-chosen location)

adequately acknowledge the social, financial, and emotional repercussions of these policies.[24] This guideline, which started from a systematic review of literature, was developed in conjunction with bioethicists and advocates for people with TB in order to integrate multiple perspectives rather than advance the traditional biomedical hierarchy. The guideline that resulted recommends that clinicians balance principles of well-being, justice, and liberty with scientific evidence and clinical expertise[24] when considering respiratory isolation. The new guidelines now ask providers and public health officers to consider proportionality, necessity, and least infringement when weighing the need for strict respiratory isolation and quarantine (**Box 1**).[24]

DISCUSSION
Barriers to Care Access and Treatment Adherence

Various barriers to TB diagnostics, linkage, and care complicate TB elimination efforts in the United States. Barriers range from individual to structural factors that are codified in laws and policy. As previously mentioned, TB transmission often occurs in lower income populations due to environmental factors like overcrowding and poor airflow, and susceptibility variables like undernutrition, alcohol use, diabetes, and HIV. However, many of the same drivers of TB infection also reduce care access. In this way, the social determinants of health create biologic vulnerability within key populations and also restrict their ability to engage in care.

Identifying individual or personal barriers to care requires intimate knowledge of an individual's life and unique circumstances. Personal finances are a key factor in care access as it influences housing and nutritional status, access to transportation, and may create concerns about treatment costs, and work disruptions.[59,60] While TB treatment in the United States is funded by the US Department of Health and Human Services and provides treatment to patients free of cost, coverage for TB prophylaxis is less clear. Private formularies may not cover preferred treatment regimens, and in the absence of universal health care, costs may accumulate for laboratory testing (IGRAs, alanine transaminase [ALT]/aspartate transaminase [AST], etc.) and management of side effects.[60] Other individual barriers to TB prevention and care include health literacy, TB self-efficacy, perceived seriousness of TB infection and TB disease, concerns about side effects, and difficulty remembering to take treatment.[61,62] In the case of TB treatment, fears about the need for quarantine and social isolation, rejection, discrimination, and status loss are acute.[63] Interpersonal barriers include perceived lack of social support from family and the medical team and anticipated, experienced or perceived social stigma toward TB that is highly stigmatized in some communities.[63,64] Finally, organizational and structural factors include regulations regarding reimbursement for adjuvant costs of testing and treatment, provider availability and accessibility, clinic locations, occupational protections like time off for diagnosis and treatment, and state and institutional policies on isolation and quarantine. These factors overlap and reify one another, further marginalizing key groups (**Table 1**).

SUMMARY

TB remains an ongoing threat globally and within the United States. Although TB disease requires exposure to *Mtb*, disease development is also driven by the infectiousness of the person with TB, host susceptibility, and the surrounding environment. The US TB Elimination Strategy underscores the need for increased provider awareness about the epidemiology of TB and prevention and treatment strategies. The CDC funds a robust educational support system for clinicians in need of ongoing education and training through the Centers of TB Excellence that complement current guidelines from the CDC, the National TB Coalition of America and the Infectious Disease Society of America. Increased contact identification, linkage, and treatment will aid in our pathway to a TB-free North America; however, to address racial, ethnic, and socioeconomic barriers in TB care, nurses, and health care workers in practice, research and policy settings must address individual, interpersonal, and organizational barriers to care and ongoing treatment adherence.

CLINICS CARE POINTS

- TB remains a significant threat to public health in the United States disproportionately burdening marginalized and vulnerable communities.
- There are 4 TB Centers of Excellence funded through the Centers for Disease Control that offer resources and support to health care workers who would like additional TB education, resources, and clinical consultation.
- TST and IGRA are 2 effective and accessible tests for effective TB screening; each has benefits and should be selected based on the client's situation.
- There are 3 recommended regimens for TB prophylaxis that should be offered to people with identified TB infection that has not progressed to TB disease.
- HPMZ is a 4 month regimen of rifapentine-moxifloxacin regimen recently approved for treatment of drug-susceptible pulmonary TB, shortening treatment by 2 months.
- The Infectious Disease Society of America has published new guidance for isolation to reduce community TB transmission; using new evidence and a person-centered lens, these guidelines prioritize least restrictive means to reduce transmission while mitigating the psychological and social impacts of isolation.

DISCLOSURES

The authors have nothing to disclose.

FUNDING

Alanna Bergman has no active funding. Tania Thomas research is supported by the National Institute of Allergy and Infectious Disease (R21AI172637).

REFERENCES

1. Global tuberculosis report. Geneva: World Health Organization; 2023.
2. Williams PM, Pratt RH, Walker WL, et al. Tuberculosis — United States, 2023. MMWR Morb Mortal Wkly Rep 2024;73(12):265–70.
3. New York City Department of Health and Mental Hygiene. Bureau of tuberculosis control annual summary, 2023, 2024.
4. Wortham JM, Haddad MB, Stewart RJ, et al. Second nationwide tuberculosis outbreak caused by bone allografts containing live cells — United States, 2023. MMWR Morb Mortal Wkly Rep 2024;72(5253):1385–9.
5. Schildknecht KR. Tuberculosis — United States, 2022. MMWR Morb Mortal Wkly Rep 2023;72. https://doi.org/10.15585/mmwr.mm7212a1.
6. Self JL, McDaniel CJ, Bamrah Morris S, et al. Estimating and evaluating tuberculosis incidence rates among people experiencing homelessness, United States, 2007–2016. Med Care 2021;59:S175.
7. Beavers SF, Pascopella L, Davidow AL, et al. Tuberculosis mortality in the United States: epidemiology and prevention opportunities. Annals ATS 2018;15(6): 683–92.
8. Centers for Disease Control and Prevention. Division of tuberculosis elimination, national center for HIV, viral hepatitis, STD and TB prevention. 2021 State and City TB Report 2022. Available at: https://www.cdc.gov/tb/statistics/indicators/2021/incidence.htm. Accessed May 21, 2024.
9. Global strategy and targets for tuberculosis prevention, care and control after 2015: report by the Secretariat. 2013. Available at: https://apps.who.int/gb/ebwha/pdf_files/eb134/b134_12-en.pdf.
10. Sakula A. Robert Koch: centenary of the discovery of the tubercle bacillus, 1882. Thorax 1928;37:246–51.
11. Daley CL, Iaccarino JM, Lange C, et al. Treatment of nontuberculous mycobacterial pulmonary disease: an official ATS/ERS/ESCMID/IDSA clinical practice guideline. Clin Infect Dis 2020;71(4):e1–36.
12. Riley RL. Airborne infection. Am J Med 1974;57(3):466–75.
13. Riley RL, Mills CC, Nyka W, et al. Aerial dissemination of pulmonary tuberculosis: a two-year study of contagion in a tuberculosis ward. Am J Epidemiol 1995; 142(1):3–14.
14. Loudon RG, Roberts RM. Singing and the dissemination of tuberculosis. Am Rev Respir Dis 1968;98(2):297–300.
15. Dinkele R, Gessner S, McKerry A, et al. Aerosolization of Mycobacterium tuberculosis by tidal breathing. Am J Respir Crit Care Med 2022;206(2):206–16.
16. Williams CM, Abdulwhhab M, Birring SS, et al. Exhaled Mycobacterium tuberculosis output and detection of subclinical disease by face-mask sampling: prospective observational studies. Lancet Infect Dis 2020;20(5):607–17.
17. Silva Miranda M, Breiman A, Allain S, et al. The tuberculous granuloma: an unsuccessful host defence mechanism providing a safety shelter for the bacteria? Clin Dev Immunol 2012;2012:1–14.
18. Rubin EJ. The granuloma in tuberculosis — friend or foe? N Engl J Med 2009; 360(23):2471–3.
19. Mathema B, Andrews JR, Cohen T, et al. Drivers of tuberculosis transmission. J Infect Dis 2017;216(suppl_6):S644–53.
20. Schurr E. Is susceptibility to tuberculosis acquired or inherited? J Intern Med 2007;261(2):106–11.

21. Ghanavi J, Farnia P, Farnia P, et al. Human genetic background in susceptibility to tuberculosis. Int J Mycobacteriol 2020;9(3):239.

22. Sinha P, Davis J, Saag L, et al. Undernutrition and tuberculosis: public health implications. J Infect Dis 2019;219(9):1356–63.

23. Bhargava A, Bhargava M, Meher A, et al. Nutritional support for adult patients with microbiologically confirmed pulmonary tuberculosis: outcomes in a programmatic cohort nested within the RATIONS trial in Jharkhand, India. Lancet Global Health 2023;11(9):e1402–11.

24. Shah M, Dansky Z, Nathavitharana R, et al. National tuberculosis coalition of America (NTCA) guidelines for respiratory isolation and restrictions to reduce transmission of pulmonary tuberculosis in community settings. Clin Infect Dis 2024;18:ciae199. https://doi.org/10.1093/cid/ciae199. Published online April.

25. Melsew YA, Doan TN, Gambhir M, et al. Risk factors for infectiousness of patients with tuberculosis: a systematic review and meta-analysis. Epidemiol Infect 2018; 146(3):345–53.

26. Urbanowski ME, Ordonez AA, Ruiz-Bedoya CA, et al. Cavitary tuberculosis: the gateway of disease transmission. Lancet Infect Dis 2020;20(6):e117–28.

27. Rouillon A, Perdrizet S, Parrot R. Transmission of tubercle bacilli: the effects of chemotherapy. Tubercle 1976;57(4):275–99.

28. Jones-López EC, Namugga O, Mumbowa F, et al. Cough aerosols of Mycobacterium tuberculosis predict new infection. A household contact study. Am J Respir Crit Care Med 2013;187(9):1007–15.

29. Fennelly KP, Jones-López EC, Ayakaka I, et al. Variability of infectious aerosols produced during coughing by patients with pulmonary tuberculosis. Am J Respir Crit Care Med 2012;186(5):450–7.

30. Theron G, Limberis J, Venter R, et al. Bacterial and host determinants of cough aerosol culture positivity in patients with drug-resistant versus drug-susceptible tuberculosis. Nat Med 2020;26(9):1435–43.

31. Dharmadhikari AS, Mphahlele M, Venter K, et al. Rapid impact of effective treatment on transmission of multidrug-resistant tuberculosis. Int J Tubercul Lung Dis 2014;18(9):1019–25.

32. Jensen PA, Lambert LA, Iademarco MF, et al. Guidelines for preventing the transmission of Mycobacterium tuberculosis in health-care settings. 2005. Available at: https://www.cdc.gov/mmwr/preview/mmwrhtml/rr5417a1.htm?s_cid=rr5417a1_e.

33. Andrews JR, Morrow C, Walensky RP, et al. Integrating social contact and environmental data in evaluating tuberculosis transmission in a South African township. J Infect Dis 2014;210(4):597–603.

34. Beijer U, Wolf A, Fazel S. Prevalence of tuberculosis, hepatitis C virus, and HIV in homeless people: a systematic review and meta-analysis. Lancet Infect Dis 2012; 12(11):859–70.

35. Baussano I, Williams BG, Nunn P, et al. Tuberculosis incidence in prisons: a systematic review. In: Menzies D, editor. PLoS Med 2010;7(12):e1000381.

36. Dara M, Acosta CD, Melchers NVSV, et al. Tuberculosis control in prisons: current situation and research gaps. Int J Infect Dis 2015;32:111–7.

37. Glynn JR, Guerra-Assunção JA, Houben RMGJ, et al. Whole genome sequencing shows a low proportion of tuberculosis disease is attributable to known close contacts in rural Malawi. In: Cardona PJ, editor. PLoS One 2015;10(7):e0132840.

38. Middelkoop K, Mathema B, Myer L, et al. Transmission of tuberculosis in a South African community with a high prevalence of HIV infection. J Infect Dis 2015; 211(1):53–61.

39. Lewinsohn DM, Leonard MK, LoBue PA, et al. Official American thoracic society/ infectious diseases society of America/centers for disease control and prevention clinical practice guidelines: diagnosis of tuberculosis in adults and children. Clin Infect Dis 2017;64(2):e1–33.

40. Kendall EA, Shrestha S, Dowdy DW. The epidemiological importance of subclinical tuberculosis. A critical reappraisal. Am J Respir Crit Care Med 2021;203(2): 168–74.

41. Drain PK, Bajema KL, Dowdy D, et al. Incipient and subclinical tuberculosis: a clinical review of early stages and progression of infection. Clin Microbiol Rev 2018;31(4):e0002118.

42. Migliori GB, Ong CWM, Petrone L, et al. The definition of tuberculosis infection based on the spectrum of tuberculosis disease. Breathe 2021;17(3):210079.

43. Esmail H, Macpherson L, Coussens AK, et al. Mind the gap – managing tuberculosis across the disease spectrum. EBioMedicine 2022;78:103928.

44. Mirzazadeh A, Kahn JG, Haddad MB, et al. State-level prevalence estimates of latent tuberculosis infection in the United States by medical risk factors, demographic characteristics and nativity. In: Quinn F, editor. PLoS One 2021;16(4): e0249012.

45. Centers for Disease Control and Prevention. Clinical testing and diagnosis for tuberculosis. 2024. Available at: https://www.cdc.gov/tb/hcp/testing-diagnosis/index.html.

46. Ayers T, Hill AN, Raykin J, et al. Comparison of tuberculin skin testing and interferon-γ release assays in predicting tuberculosis disease. JAMA Netw Open 2024;7(4):e244769.

47. QuantiFERON. FAQs for health professionals: QuantiFERON®-TB gold. 2020. Available at: https://www.quantiferon.com/wp-content/uploads/2017/05/PROM-10157_FAQs-Health-Professionals-Rev001v02.pdf.

48. Tuberculosis. In: Kimberlin DW, Banerjee R, Barnett ED, et al, editors. Red book: 2024–2027 report of the committee on infectious diseases. 33rd edition. Itasca (IL): American Academy of Pediatrics; 2024. p. 888–920.

49. Turner NA, Ahmed A, Haley CA, et al. Use of interferon-gamma release assays in children <2 Years old. Journal of the Pediatric Infectious Diseases Society 2023; 12(8):481–5.

50. Sterling TR, Njie G, Zenner D, et al. Guidelines for the treatment of latent tuberculosis infection: recommendations from the national tuberculosis controllers association and CDC, 2020. MMWR Recomm Rep (Morb Mortal Wkly Rep) 2020; 69(1):1–11.

51. Nahid P, Dorman SE, Alipanah N, et al. Official American thoracic society/centers for disease control and prevention/infectious diseases society of America clinical practice guidelines: treatment of drug-susceptible tuberculosis. Clin Infect Dis 2016. https://doi.org/10.1093/cid/ciw566.

52. Carr W, Kurbatova E, Starks A, et al. Interim guidance: 4-month rifapentine-moxifloxacin regimen for the treatment of drug-susceptible pulmonary tuberculosis — United States, 2022. MMWR Morb Mortal Wkly Rep 2022;71(8):285–9.

53. Dorman SE, Nahid P, Kurbatova EV, et al. Four-month rifapentine regimens with or without moxifloxacin for tuberculosis. N Engl J Med 2021;384(18):1705–18.

54. Arcangelo VP, Peterson AM, Wilbur VF, et al. Pharmacotherapeutics for advanced practice. 5th edition. Philadelphia, PA: Wolters Kluwer; 2022.

55. Lew W, Pai M, Oxlade O, et al. Initial drug resistance and tuberculosis treatment outcomes: systematic review and meta-analysis. Ann Intern Med 2008; 149(2):123.

56. Division of tuberculosis elimination, national center for HIV, viral hepatitis, STD, and TB prevention, centers for disease control and prevention. Reported tuberculosis in the United States, 2022. 2022. Available at: https://www.cdc.gov/tb/statistics/reports/2022/Exec_Commentary.html#conclusion.

57. Cox HS, Niemann S, Ismailov G, et al. Risk of acquired drug resistance during short-course directly observed treatment of tuberculosis in an area with high levels of drug resistance. Clin Infect Dis 2007;44(11):1421–7.

58. Mangan JM, Woodruff RS, Winston CA, et al. Recommendations for use of video directly observed therapy during tuberculosis treatment — United States, 2023. MMWR Morb Mortal Wkly Rep 2023;72(12):313–6.

59. Joseph HA, Shrestha-Kuwahara R, Lowry D, et al. Factors influencing health care workers' adherence to work site tuberculosis screening and treatment policies. Am J Infect Control 2004;32(8):456–61.

60. Liu Y, Birch S, Newbold KB, et al. Barriers to treatment adherence for individuals with latent tuberculosis infection: a systematic search and narrative synthesis of the literature. Int J Health Plann Manag 2018;33(2):e416–33.

61. Spence BC, Bruxvoort K, Munoz-Plaza C, et al. Patient-reported barriers to treatment initiation and completion for latent tuberculosis infection among patients within a large integrated health care system in southern California. J Publ Health Manag Pract 2023;29(3):345–52.

62. Hirsch-Moverman Y, Shrestha-Kuwahara R, Bethel J, et al. Latent tuberculous infection in the United States and Canada: who completes treatment and why? Int J Tubercul Lung Dis 2015;19(1):31–8.

63. Moya EM, Lusk MW. Tuberculosis stigma and perceptions in the US-Mexico border. Salud Publica Mex 2013;55(Supl.4):498.

64. Royce RA, Colson PW, Woodsong C, et al, For the Tuberculosis Epidemiologic Studies Consortium (TBESC). Tuberculosis knowledge, awareness, and stigma among African-Americans in three southeastern counties in the USA: a qualitative study of community perspectives. J Racial and Ethnic Health Disparities 2017;4(1):47–58.

Chronic Hepatitis C Infection
Is Elimination a Myth or in Our Midst?

Check for updates

Sherilyn Camille Brinkley, BA, BSN, MSN, NP

KEYWORDS

- Chronic hepatitis C • Simplified treatment • Direct acting antivirals
- Elimination plans • Barriers to care

KEY POINTS

- Rates of chronic Hepatitis C virus (HCV) are on the rise in the United States despite the availability of safe, well-tolerated, curative treatments.
- Untreated HCV can lead to progressive liver disease including cirrhosis, hepatocellular carcinoma (HCC), and the need for transplantation.
- Expanded screening guidelines, highly effective oral therapies, simplified treatment algorithms, and improved diagnostic tests offer the rare opportunity to eliminate HCV worldwide.
- Multiple barriers to HCV screening, diagnosis and treatment exist and the expansion of low-threshold services among nonspecialist providers is necessary to increase treatment uptake.
- There are national and international HCV elimination proposals in place but a comprehensive, federally funded program has not been implemented and requires significant political and public health investment to see it through.

INTRODUCTION

Hepatitis C virus (HCV) infection remains a disease of global concern and a major cause of liver cirrhosis, HCC and liver transplantation. Despite the availability of highly efficacious direct-acting antiviral agents (DAAs) with cure rates greater than 95% in just 8 to 12 weeks, the majority of the estimated 71 million persons living with HCV worldwide remain untreated and the burden is expected to grow. In the United States, recent estimates indicate that the number of people currently living with HCV is approximately 4 million making HCV the most common blood-borne infectious disease.[1] It is associated with significant morbidity and mortality contributing to approximately 14,000 deaths per year with deaths higher for Black people (5 per 100,000) and Hispanic people (4 per 100,000) than for White people (3 per 100,000).[2] Infection with HCV is typically associated with substance use, mental health disorders, and

Funding Support: Non-CME speaking fees from Gilead Sciences and AbbVie.
Johns Hopkins University, Division of Infectious Diseases, 725 North Wolfe Street, Fisher Center 218, Baltimore, MD 21205, USA
E-mail address: sbrinkle@jhmi.edu

Nurs Clin N Am 60 (2025) 507–522
https://doi.org/10.1016/j.cnur.2024.10.009
0029-6465/25/© 2024 Elsevier Inc. All rights reserved, including those for text and data mining, AI training, and similar technologies.

low-income populations driving barriers of stigma and discrimination that ultimately impact care engagement. The steady rise in new HCV infections among people who inject drugs (PWID) has led to the evolution of 2 distinct groups living with HCV in the United States: (1) An older cohort largely infected through unsafe medical practices from the past, many of whom have comorbidities including obesity, alcohol use, and diabetes placing them at higher risk for cirrhosis; and (2) A younger group with recent HCV acquisition driven largely by injection drug use (IDU) practices.[3] The expansion of HCV screening guidelines, the development of innovative diagnostics, and the evolution of simplified treatment modalities have not overcome the new and persistent challenges that mark the US viral hepatitis landscape. In 2023, the White House proposed a comprehensive National HCV Elimination Plan which awaits Congressional approval, fund allocation, and implementation. The critical need for the health care community, public health advocates, and Congress to partner in the realization of a well-funded elimination plan is long overdue. Steadfast efforts to reduce barriers to diagnosis and treatment are paramount to halt the downstream morbidity and mortality of untreated HCV. This article will explore the current HCV disease burden in the United States, sources of transmission, recommendations for HCV screening, evaluation, and treatment, including obstacles to cure and strategies underway to advance elimination goals.

BACKGROUND

Hepatitis describes liver inflammation, which can originate from various sources including viruses such as hepatitis A, B, C, D or E, drugs, chemicals, alcohol, autoimmune conditions, complications of pregnancy, liver steatosis, or genetic disorders. HCV is a viral infection causing both acute and chronic hepatitis with a disease severity range between mild, asymptomatic illness to severe life-threatening liver disease. First described as non-A, non-B hepatitis in the 1970s, it was in 1989 that this blood-borne pathogen was identified and named as hepatitis C virus. Most individuals with new or acute HCV infection do not have a clinically evident illness and may not seek medical attention. This has contributed to approximately 50% of all infected persons remaining unaware that they have HCV infection.[4-7]

Around 30% (15%–45%) of newly infected persons spontaneously clear the virus within 6 months of the exposure. Approximately 70% (55%–85%) of those exposed to HCV will develop chronic infection or persistent HCV RNA, the ribonucleic acid (RNA) of the HCV, thus requiring treatment for eradication. There have been challenges in tracking HCV infection rates, and for each acute HCV case reported in the United States, the Center for Disease Control and Prevention (CDC) estimates approximately 13.9 actual new HCV cases occurred.[8,9] For example, in 2021, a total of 5023 new cases of acute HCV were reported to the CDC; based on this number, the CDC estimated 69,800 new cases of HCV in 2021.[8] New infections have increased steadily since 2014 driven by the opioid epidemic with increased injection drug use practices among a younger cohort.[8] By 2022, following over a decade of consecutive annual increases in acute HCV, the number of acute HCV cases declined for the first time. During 2022, a total of 4848 acute cases were reported, corresponding to 67,400 estimated infections after adjusting for case underascertainment and underreporting. The number of cases reported during 2022 corresponded to a 3.5% decrease from the 5023 cases reported during 2021 and a 99% increase from the 2436 cases reported during 2015[9] (Fig. 1).

The 2013 to 2016 National Health and Nutrition Examination Survey (NHANES) gathered data among the general noninstitutionalized US population reflecting an estimated 4.1 million people to have had HCV exposure (HCV antibody positive) including

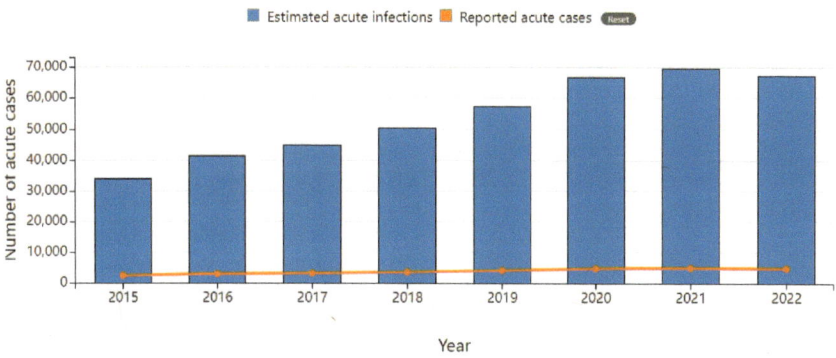

Fig. 1. Number of reported cases and estimated infections of acute hepatitis C- United States, 2015 to 2022. The number of estimated viral hepatitis infections was determined by multiplying the number of reported cases that met the classification criteria for a confirmed case by a factor that adjusted for underascertainment and underreporting. (*Data from*: CDC, National Notifiable Diseases Surveillance System. https://www.cdc.gov/hepatitis/statistics/2022surveillance/hepatitis-c/figure-3.1.htm#print.)

2.4 million with active HCV RNA in the bloodstream.[1] The total US burden of disease however includes those not accounted for in the NHANES study including incarcerated, institutionalized, and unsheltered homeless individuals, which adds an estimated 380,000 to 800,000 additional HCV exposed individuals.[1,10] A separate analysis to account for populations inadequately represented in NHANES found that despite years of an effective cure, the prevalence of HCV in 2017 to 2020 remains unchanged from 2013 to 2016 when using comparable methodology. This translates into an estimated HCV RNA prevalence of 1.0% among the US adults in 2017 to 2020, corresponding to 2,463,700 current infections when using the NHANES model of analysis. A separate model that accounts for the rising rates of HCV among PWID, estimates the HCV RNA prevalence to be 1.6% corresponding to 4,043,200 current infections.[11]

BURDEN OF DISEASE

Hepatitis C is a small, single-stranded, enveloped RNA virus with a high degree of genetic heterogeneity that infects the liver. Seven distinct HCV genotypes have been identified worldwide with genotype 1 being the most prevalent in the United States accounting for approximately 75% of cases.[11,12] Unlike hepatitis A and hepatitis B, there is no vaccine available to prevent HCV and if left untreated, HCV can lead to progressive liver disease. The risk of progression to cirrhosis, a widespread deposition of scar tissue in the liver, ranges from 10% to 20% within the first 20 to 30 years of exposure.[12] There are extrahepatic manifestations of HCV involving almost every organ system in the body contributing to metabolic syndromes, autoimmune conditions, malignancy, dermatologic conditions, renal disease, psychiatric disease, and immune-mediated disorders such as mixed cryoglobulinemia.[13] In 2017, people living with HCV died at a median age of 61 years, approximately 18 years younger than the average lifespan in the United States.[14,15]

TRANSMISSION

As the most common blood-borne infection in the United States, HCV is primarily spread through percutaneous exposure to infected blood. At least 60% of acute infections in the Unites States result from injection drug use practices. Transmission often occurs through shared needles, syringes, or other paraphernalia used to prepare and inject drugs. Other modes of transmission include tattoos performed in unregulated tattoo settings such as jails or prisons, and contaminated supplies shared for noninjection drug use. Sexual transmission may occur but is not an efficient means of viral spread except among human immunodeficiency virus (HIV)-infected men who have unprotected sex with other men.[16] Healthcare exposures have been another route of transmission including the receipt of blood products in the United States prior to 1992; receipt of clotting factor concentrates in the United States before 1987; receipt of blood or blood products in other countries; long-term hemodialysis; needlestick injuries among healthcare workers; patient to patient transmission resulting from poor infection control practices.[17] Because of the increasing incidence of HCV infection among women of childbearing age, perinatal transmission (intrauterine or intrapartum) has become an increasingly important mode of HCV transmission.[18,19] HCV positivity increased by 39 % among pregnant women from 2011 to 2016.[15] A systematic review and meta-analysis of studies conducted in multiple countries shows a 5.8% risk for perinatal transmission among infants born to HCV-infected mothers with double the rate of transmission to infants born from HCV and HIV coinfected women.[20]

HEPATITIS C VIRUS SCREENING AMONG ADULTS

HCV screening is recommended because of the established benefits of treatment in reducing the risk of decompensated cirrhosis, hepatocellular carcinoma, and all-cause mortality. Early detection and treatment can prevent serious liver damage to improve long-term health outcomes and prevent transmission to others. In 2020, the CDC and the US Preventative Services Task Force expanded HCV screening recommendations for adolescents and adults as this was deemed cost-effective because of increasing incidence and prevalence among PWID and the decreasing cost of treatment with DAA.[10,21] The new recommendations updated routine HCV screening to include one-time HCV antibody testing (HCV Ab) for individuals 18 years and older (**Table 1**). Individuals at risk of repeat HCV exposure should have testing completed more frequently. The presence of HCV antibodies is not protective against reinfection and therefore repeat exposure to HCV could lead to new infection.

The two-step process for HCV screening and diagnosis includes an initial HCV Ab test, which can be a laboratory-based assay or a point-of-care (POCT) assay, followed by a confirmatory HCV RNA, a blood test that detects the presence of hepatitis C virus in the blood used to confirm active infection. A positive HCV Ab result could reflect one of the 3 scenarios: (1) Current HCV infection, (2) Past HCV infection, or (3) Biologic false positive antibody consistent with no infection. A positive HCV Ab test reflects HCV exposure but does not indicate active infection. For example, individuals who have a positive HCV Ab test and a negative HCV RNA result do not have laboratory evidence of current HCV infection. This suggests HCV RNA clearance at the time of exposure or past HCV treatment with viral elimination (**Fig. 2**). The HCV Ab test becomes positive within 8 to 11 weeks of the initial HCV exposure whereas HCV RNA is present in the blood 1 to 2 weeks following new infection. The preferred approach to HCV screening using traditional phlebotomy consists of an HCV Ab test with an automatic reflex step to the HCV RNA test among HCV Ab reactive samples. This affords one blood draw only to diagnose active HCV infection. The HCV Ab POCT and

Table 1
Recommendations for one-time Hepatitis C testing

Recommended	Rating[a]
One-time, routine, opt out HCV testing is recommended for all individuals aged 18 y or older.	I, B
One-time HCV testing should be performed for all persons <18 year old with activities, exposures, or conditions or circumstances associated with an increased risk of HCV infection (see below).	I, B
Prenatal HCV testing as part of routine prenatal care is recommended with each pregnancy.	I, B
Periodic repeat HCV testing should be offered to all persons with activities, exposures, or conditions or circumstances associated with an increased risk of HCV exposure (see below).	IIa, C
Annual HCV testing is recommended for all PWID, for HIV-infected men who have unprotected sex with men, and men who have sex with men taking preexposure prophylaxis (PrEP).	IIa, C

Risk Activities
- Injection drug use (current or ever, including those who injected only once)
- Intranasal illicit drug use
- Use of glass crack pipes
- Male engagement in sex with men
- Engagement in chem sex (defined as the intentional combining of sex with the use of particular nonprescription drugs in order to facilitate or enhance the sexual encounter[47])

Risk Exposures
- Persons on long-term hemodialysis (ever)
- Persons with percutaneous/parenteral exposures in an unregulated setting
- Healthcare, emergency medical, and public safety workers after needlestick, sharps, or mucosal exposure to HCV-infected blood
- Children born to HCV-infected women
- Recipients of a prior transfusion or organ transplant, including persons who:
  ○ Were notified that they received blood from a donor who later tested positive for HCV
  ○ Received a transfusion of blood or blood components, or underwent an organ transplant before July 1992
  ○ Received clotting factor concentrates produced before 1987
- Persons who were ever incarcerated

Other Conditions and Circumstances
- HIV or HBV infection
- Sexually active persons about to start PrEP for HIV
- Chronic liver disease and/or chronic hepatitis, including unexplained elevated ALTlevels
- Solid organ donors (living and deceased) and solid organ transplant recipients

Abbreviations: ALT, alanine aminotransferase; PrEP, preexposure prophylaxis.
  [a] Please refer to https://www.hcvguidelines.org/contents/methods/table-2.
  From HCV Guidance: Recommendations for Testing, Managing, and Treating Hepatitis C; with permission. AASLD and IDSA. HCV Guidance: Recommendations for Testing, Managing, and Treating Hepatitis C. 2024. Available at: https://www.hcvguidelines.org/evaluate/testing-and-linkage Accessed October 1, 2024.

HCV RNA POCT assays allow for a finger stick sample rather than standard phlebotomythat affords convenient testing in community settings to capture individuals less engaged in routine medical care. The Food and Drug Administration (FDA)-approved HCV Ab POCT takes 20 minutes to result and could be immediately followed by the HCV RNA POCT that offers a qualitative result within approximately 1 hour of sample collection. Diagnostic advancements in POCT options offer increased flexibilities to reach marginalized groups located in nonclinical or rural settings or those without

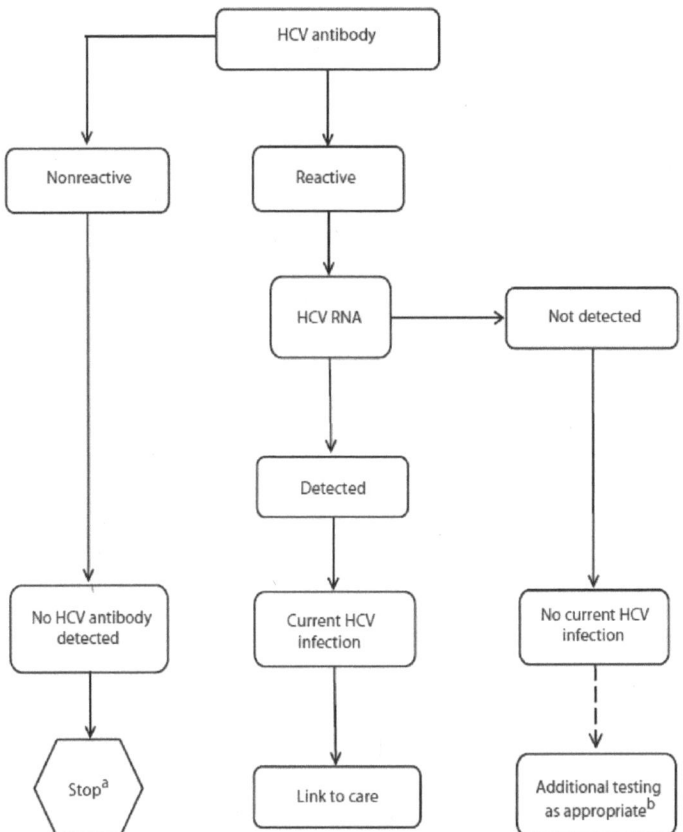

Fig. 2. CDC- recommended testing sequence for identifying current HCV infection. [a]For persons who might have been exposed to HCV within the past 6 months, testing for HCV RNA or follow-up testing for HCV antibody is recommended. For persons who are immunocompromised, testing for HCV RNA can be considered. [b]To differentiate past, resolved HCV infection from biologic false positivity for HCV antibody, testing with another HCV antibody assay can be considered. Repeat HCV RNA testing if the person tested is suspected to have had HCV exposure within the past 6 months or has clinical evidence of HCV disease, or if there is concern regarding the handling or storage of the test specimen. (*Data from* Centers for Disease Control and Prevention (CDC). Testing for HCV infection: an update of guidance for clinicians and laboratorians. MMWR Morb Mortal Wkly Rep. 2013 May 10;62(18):362-365.)

medical insurance coverage, low-income individuals, the disabled, senior citizens, persons who use drugs, and unsheltered individuals. An innovative HCV core antigen test is in the diagnostic pipeline and will enable a one-step diagnosis of active HCV in the future.

HEPATITIS C VIRUS SCREENING AMONG INFANTS AND CHILDREN

In 2023, the CDC modified recommendations for testing HCV among perinatally exposed infants and children. In these guidelines, perinatally exposed infants and children are those born to pregnant persons with current HCV RNA positivity during pregnancy or those with probable HCV infection based on a reactive HCV Ab test with no confirmatory HCV RNA result. Rates of chronic HCV among persons of childbearing age have risen substantially over the past 2 decades and routine HCV screening is now recommended during each pregnancy. For perinatally exposed infants and children, the CDC recommends the following:

- HCV RNA testing at age 2 to 6 months: Note, no further follow-up is needed after a negative HCV RNA that is performed at age 2 to 6 months, unless clinically warranted (ie, clinical symptoms or signs or laboratory findings are consistent with hepatitis C).
- Infants and children with a positive HCV RNA test should be managed in consultation with a provider experienced in pediatric HCV management.
- Infants and children with undetectable HCV RNA do not have a current HCV infection and do not require further testing.
- Infants and children 7 to 17 months of age who were not previously tested should undergo HCV RNA testing.
- Children 18 months of age and older who were not previously tested should undergo HCV Ab testing with reflexive HCV RNA.[22]

LINKAGE TO HEPATITIS C VIRUS CARE GAPS

Many individuals diagnosed with HCV infection do not get linked to care and treatment.[5] Several reasons for linkage gaps have been reported including failure of medical providers to make a referral, lack of medical insurance, lack of transportation services, substance use, mental health disorders, housing instability, or fear of stigma.[23] Potential strategies to improve linkage to care include decentralizing treatment by colocating services in primary care, mobile units, syringe services programs, and addiction treatment facilities; incorporating Peer Navigator and Care Coordinator services to support insurance acquisition, transportation, linkage, and retention in care; and contingency management, a type of behavioral therapy to reinforce a positive behavioral change with incentivization or reward.[24] One novel program leveraged onsite HCV telemedicine services to persons enrolled in addiction treatment programs versus standard referral to an outside specialist. Opioid treatment program-integrated telemedicine resulted in significantly higher HCV cure rates compared with off-site referral, with high participant satisfaction. Illicit drug use declined significantly among cured participants with minimal reinfections.[25] This is one example of a strategy to enhance access to HCV treatment services through low-threshold linkage to care designed to meet persons living with HCV in a familiar, nonstigmatizing environment.

PRETREATMENT EVALUATION

The American Association for the Study of Liver Diseases (AASLD) and the Infectious Diseases Society of America (IDSA) have joined to create a guidance document with frequent updates pending new information and treatments. HCV guidance: Recommendations for testing, managing, and treating Hepatitis C is an evolving report that is accessed online to obtain the most current information about how to manage and treat persons with HCV infection.[17] The individual who presents to care with HCV infection could be newly diagnosed or previously diagnosed ready to establish care. Regardless of the duration of infection, HCV treatment is recommended with rare exception. According to AASLD-IDSA HCV Guidelines, "Treatment is recommended for all patients with acute or chronic HCV infection except those with a short life expectancy that cannot be remediated by HCV therapy, liver transplantation, or another directed therapy. Patients with a short life expectancy owing to liver disease should be managed in consultation with an expert".[17] The goal of HCV therapy is a sustained virologic response (SVR) or virologic cure defined as the continued absence of detectable HCV RNA for at least 12 weeks after completion of therapy. Among persons who achieve cure, HCV antibodies will persist lifelong, but HCV RNA will not be detectable in the serum, and liver histology can improve over time.[26]

Evaluation of patients with chronic HCV infection focuses on assessing factors that inform antiviral selection and identifying complications and common comorbidities that may impact prognosis and other management decisions. The first step in the evaluation of HCV is to confirm the presence of a reactive HCV Ab test and detectable HCV RNA in the blood.[27] In addition, the clinician should strive to establish a therapeutic relationship with the patient to assess their understanding of the treatment goals and to provide education about the treatment process, medication adherence strategies, and harm reduction principles to avoid transmission and reinfection. A thorough history and physical examination are the foundation of the initial assessment to ascertain the following.

- Risk factors for acquiring HCV infection
- Presence of significant medical comorbidities
- Review of current medications
- Current or past substance use disorders
- Coinfection with other blood-borne viruses (eg, HIV, hepatitis B virus [HBV])
- Stigmata of chronic liver disease
- Clinical manifestations attributable to HCV infection
- A history of prior HCV treatment
- Housing stability
- Willingness to proceed with treatment[28]

Counseling points to reinforce during the initial and subsequent encounters include education aimed at reducing liver disease progression and preventing HCV transmission.

- Eat a well-balanced diet.
- Exercise regularly.
- Avoid excessive alcohol intake with the goal of abstinence
- Talk to your clinician before taking prescription drugs, herbal products, or nutritional supplements
- Update your clinician on current medications, supplements, and over-the-counter drugs at each encounter
- Get tested for HIV and hepatitis B
- Get vaccinated against hepatitis A and hepatitis B.
- Consider moderate to high coffee consumption to benefit the liver
- Avoid sharing items contaminated with blood such as personal care items, supplies used to prepare or inject drugs
- Avoid unprotected sexual encounters with persons known to have HIV[28]

A key component of the pretreatment assessment is a liver fibrosis measurement to predict HCV liver disease progression and to guide management decisions. Hepatic fibrosis is a dynamic scarring process and a precursor to cirrhosis. Evaluation for fibrosis using noninvasive blood markers, liver elastography, and rarely a liver biopsy, is recommended to facilitate appropriate choice in HCV treatment and to determine the need to initiate measures for the management of cirrhosis long term. Individuals with severe fibrosis or cirrhosis require surveillance monitoring for liver cancer, esophageal varices, and liver function long term.[17] In cases where commercial serologic markers or liver elastography are not available to assess the degree of fibrosis, the AST-to-platelet ratio index https://www.hepatitisc.uw.edu/page/clinical-calculators/apri or FIB-4 index score https://www.hepatitisc.uw.edu/page/clinical-calculators/fib-4 can prove helpful but neither is sensitive enough to rule out advanced fibrosis.[29] These require a limited number of variables to calculate a result that may be used to predict disease severity and to guide treatment decisions.

In addition to a liver fibrosis assessment, Hepatitis B screening tests should be completed during the HCV pretreatment phase. Because reactivation of HBV, in some cases with fulminant hepatitis, has been reported in rare patients receiving HCV DAA therapy, all patients should undergo testing for HBV coinfection with 3 serologic markers prior to initiation of HCV therapy (**Table 2**). Hepatology, gastroenterology, or infectious disease specialists should be consulted for guidance on HBV management and consideration of HBV antiviral treatment among HBV/HCV coinfected individuals prior to the start of HCV antivirals. The AASLD-IDSA Guidelines should be referenced for the complete pretreatment work-up as well as on-treatment and posttreatment monitoring recommendations for a variety of HCV patient types. Pretreatment screening for drug-drug interactions with the selected HCV DAA is completed by consulting the prescribing information, a pharmacist, AASLD-IDSA HCV Guidelines, or University of Liverpool drug interaction checker: http://www.hep-druginteractions.org. Education about the proper administration of the DAA regimen including dose, frequency, food effects, missed doses, adverse events, and adherence strategies should be provided during the pretreatment timeframe to prepare for a successful course of therapy.[17]

HEPATITIS C VIRUS TREATMENT

Achieving HCV cure can result in improved survival, reduced morbidity, and higher quality of life. DAA are powerful all-oral, once a day medications offering minimal adverse effects, high rates of cure, and short durations of treatment. There are DAAs available in 4 unique drug classes defined by mechanism of action and therapeutic target (**Table 3**). This article will focus on the most commonly used regimens in the United States based on the simplified approach to HCV treatment spelled out in the AASLD-IDSA guidance document. The majority living with HCV fall under the category of treatment naïve, no HIV, no Hepatitis B, no cirrhosis, or compensated cirrhosis.[17] This affords the use of a simplified treatment approach developed to streamline HCV evaluation, treatment, and posttreatment follow-up. There are 2 unique simplified HCV treatment algorithms based on the liver fibrosis assessment.

Table 2 Hepatitis B screening tests	
Hepatitis B Serologic Markers	**Description**
HBsAg	Protein on surface of HBV detected during acute or chronic HBV infection
(Anti-HBc- total)	Indicates HBV exposure (previous or ongoing infection)
HBsAb	Indicates immunity to HBV, either through vaccination or immune clearance

Abbreviations: HBc, Hepatitis B core; HBsAb, Hepatitis B surface antibody; HBsAg, Hepatitis B surface antigen.

Data from Trepo C, Chan HLY, Lok A. Hepatitis B virus infection. Lancet 2014:384: 2053-63.

Table 3
First line Hepatitis C virus direct-acting antivirals

Classes of DAAs	Fixed-Dose Combination Regimens	Single-Drug Agents
NS5B RNA-dependent RNA polymerase inhibitors	Glecaprevir-pibrentasvir	Sofosbuvir
NS5A inhibitors	Sofosbuvir-velpatasvir	Daclatasvir
NS3/4A protease inhibitors	Ledipasvir-sofosbuvir	Simeprevir
	Sofosbuvir-velpatasvir-voxilaprevir	
	Elbasvir-grazoprevir	

Data from AASLD and IDSA. HCV Guidance: Recommendations for Testing, Managing, and Treating Hepatitis C. 2024. Available at: www.hcvguidelines.org. Accessed October 1, 2024.

1. An algorithm for treatment-naïve adults without cirrhosis: https://www.hcv guidelines.org/sites/default/files/full-guidance-pdf/AASLD-IDSA_HCV-Guidance_ TxN-Simplified-Tx-No-Cirr_e.pdf
2. An algorithm for treatment-naive adults with compensated cirrhosis: https://www. hcvguidelines.org/sites/default/files/full-guidance-pdf/AASLD-IDSA_HCV-Guidance_ TxN-Simplified-Tx-Comp-Cirr_e.pdf

Each algorithm provides a comprehensive step-by-step guide to HCV management and can be easily accessed online or printed as a PDF for reference. This consolidated approach is expected to expand the number of clinicians who prescribe DAA therapy and thus increase the number of persons treated. For initial therapy of chronic HCV infection, the AASLD-IDSA simplified treatment guidance recommends one of the following pangenotypic DAA regimens for those with no cirrhosis or compensated cirrhosis.

- *Sofosbuvir-velpatasvir:* a one pill once a day regimen for 12 weeks. This is well-tolerated with less than 1% of clinical trial participants discontinuing the regimen for adverse events. The most common adverse events are fatigue, headache, nausea, nasopharyngitis, and insomnia.[30] Several trials with sofosbuvir-velpatasvir have demonstrated very high efficacy for initial therapy of all genotypes (SVR rates 95–100%) and from real world observational data that match trial findings.[30,31]
- *Glecaprevir-pibrentasvir:* a 3 pill once a day regimen with food for 8 weeks. This regimen is well-tolerated with an analysis of pooled data from multiple clinical trials demonstrating most adverse effects to be mild, with headache and fatigue reported as the most common complaints.[32] Fewer than 0.5% of patients discontinued therapy because of adverse effects. Support for glecaprevir-pibrentasvir comes from several trials showing very high efficacy for initial therapy of all genotypes (SVR rates 95–99%) and from real world observational data that match trial findings.[33,34]

The choice between regimens is primarily limited by availability; in the United States, some payers will provide coverage for a single preferred regimen. If both are options, the choice depends on potential for drug interactions and patient preference. For those who do not qualify for the simplified treatment algorithms due to characteristics that fall outside the qualifying parameters, the AASLD-IDSA HCV Guidelines provide detailed recommendations for the approach to management and treatment of a variety of patient types and special populations including those with prior treatment experience, HIV/HCV coinfection, HBV/HCV coinfection, decompensated cirrhosis, postliver transplant, organ recipients from HCV viremic donors, kidney transplant, HCV in pregnancy, and HCV in children.

TREATMENT ACCESS

The arrival of the first all-oral, interferon-free HCV DAA regimens in 2014 revolutionized the HCV treatment landscape. DAAs interfere directly and specifically with certain viral proteins required for HCV replication resulting in a rapid and sustainable viral decline when dosed consistently and for the required duration. Antivirals from distinct classes with different modes of action are combined to prevent viral replication and delay the development of drug resistance to allow for complete viral clearance in the majority of those treated. This development was a dramatic shift from the complex therapies comprised of weekly pegylated interferon (INF) injections in combination with antiviral pills that drove significant toxicity and left many ineligible or poor candidates for treatment. Before the INF-free era, specific subpopulations including patients with HCV/HIV coinfection, those with renal impairment, obesity, cirrhosis, certain racial or ethnic backgrounds, prior treatment failure, particular HCV genotypes, or high HCV RNA viral loads had poor virologic response to treatment.[35,36] With the arrival of oral DAA combination regimens offering simplified dosing, minimal side effects, and high efficacy, the average wholesale price for a course of HCV treatment of $90,000 per course per patient posed a new challenge to treatment access. The high cost of treatment threatened payer affordability based on whether a payer had sufficient resources in the annual health care budget to cover the cost of a new therapy for all who may need or want it within that year.[17] Payers throughout the United States instituted barriers to HCV treatment access including 4 major types of restrictions adopted by many state Medicaid programs as outlined below.

1. *Fibrosis Level Treatment Restrictions:* Fibrosis restrictions require patients to wait until HCV severely damages their liver to a certain level before receiving treatment. Fibrosis is estimated on a scale from 0 to 4, with 4 indicating liver failure or cirrhosis.
2. *Sobriety Treatment Restrictions*: These restrictions require patients to abstain from using alcohol and/or drugs for a specified period of time before starting HCV treatment, or to document screening, counseling or treatment engagement before HCV treatment can begin. The period of required sobriety can range from 1 to 6 months before treatment.
3. *Prescriber Treatment Restrictions* : These restrictions limit the type of clinicians that can prescribe HCV treatment. State Medicaid programs with prescriber restrictions require consultation with a specialist, or that a specialist directly prescribes treatment, which can hinder treatment in areas with few specialists.
4. *Prior Authorization:* Prior authorization is an administrative process whereby healthcare providers must submit paperwork for approval before an insurance company will decide whether to cover a medication or service. This extra bureaucracy creates further barriers to streamlined treatment.[37]

Since the introduction of HCV treatment restrictions in 2014, the United States has made steady progress in reducing barriers to care through improved access to treatment in most states. This success has been driven by local, state, and national advocacy groups including the Center for Health Law and Policy Innovation of Harvard Law School and the National Viral Hepatitis Roundtable. Emerging data has shown the use of DAAs to be cost-effective because they curtail HCV progression, reduce risk for cirrhosis, liver failure, and hepatocellular carcinoma thus contributing to public health cost savings over time.[3] Despite these strides, the CDC released data in 2022 showing that large gaps in HCV treatment persist nearly a decade after the approval of a highly effective cure. According to the report, less than 1 in 3 people with health insurance receive DAAs within a year of diagnosis (**Fig. 3**). In addition, treatment is lowest among

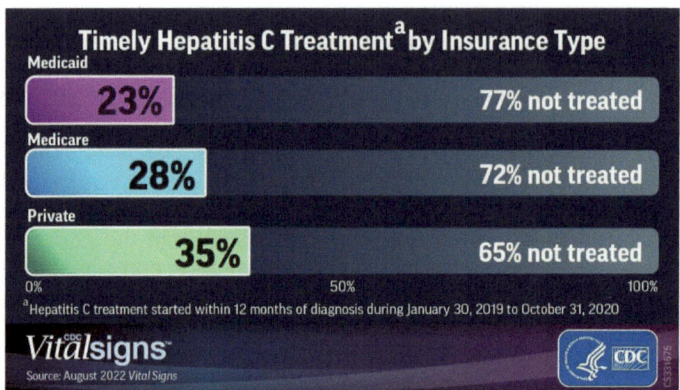

Fig. 3. Hepatitis C treatment among insured adults 2019 to 2020. (*Data from*: Thompson WW, Symum H, Sandul A, et al. Vital Signs: Hepatitis C Treatment Among Insured Adults — United States, 2019–2020. MMWR Morb Mortal Wkly Rep 2022;71:1011-1017.)

young adults aged 18 to 29 years, Medicaid recipients, persons reporting Black or other race, and those living in states with ongoing treatment restrictions.[2]

EXPANDING CLINICIAN CAPACITY

The evolution of HCV treatment in recent years has allowed a variety of healthcare professionals to cultivate HCV management skills and move HCV care outside the traditional gastroenterology, hepatology, and infectious disease specialty practice. One strategy to increase testing and treatment is the integration of HCV care into primary care settings. Innovative training programs and collaborative models to transform practice allow for expansion of the HCV treatment workforce. Programs such as the Extension for Community Healthcare Outcomes model provide group video conferencing to support new treaters in the management of HCV.[38] A similar model has been employed in the Sharing the Cure program, a public health implementation project to improve HCV treatment access through didactic instruction and case-based training of primary care providers in the management of HCV.[39] Those clinicians working in community health, addiction or carceral settings comprised of higher concentrations of persons living with untreated HCV are ideally positioned to expand HCV service delivery to lower disease burden.[40] The National Clinician Consultation Center for Hepatitis C management provides free clinician-to-clinician advice by phone 844-437 to 4636 Monday through Friday, 9 AM to 8 PM EST or by submitting an online case at the Clinician Consultation Center website.[41] In addition, the AASLD-IDSA HCV guidance and the World Health Organization (WHO) guidance on Hepatitis C offer a comprehensive resource containing current information about the simplified care of persons with HCV and a management pathway to overcome barriers in access to testing and treatment.[17,42]

UNITED STATES ELIMINATION PLAN

In 2016, the WHO declared the objective to eliminate HCV infection as a public health threat by 2030 through a plan to minimize new chronic infections and to decrease HCV-related mortality. The targets for elimination include the diagnosis of 90% of those living with chronic HCV and the treatment of 80% of those diagnosed in conjunction with interventions to curb transmission of HCV among high-risk groups.[43]

The Division of Viral Hepatitis at the Centers for Disease Control and Prevention issued a 2025 strategic plan for HCV elimination that outlines the following goals for 2025 and 2030 when compared to a baseline in 2017.[44]

- Decrease new HCV infections by 22% for 2025 and by 90% for 2030
- Reduce HCV-related death rate by 27% for 2025 and by 65% for 2030
- Reduce rate of new HCV infections in persons who inject drugs by 26% for 2025 and by 90% for 2030
- Increase proportion of persons with HCV viral clearance by 35% for 2025 and by 86% for 2030[43]

These elimination goals have proved challenging amid the ongoing opioid epidemic in the United States with an overall 106% increase in the estimated number of new HCV infections from 2015 to 2021.[8] Multilevel barriers at the patient, clinician, and system levels contribute to the difficulties with access to HCV testing and treatment. The mission to eliminate HCV will require not only improved access to diagnostics and treatments but an unwavering commitment to work with a broad range of partners at the national and community level. This requires the continued revision and removal of policies that restrict access to viral hepatitis services, the promotion of outreach to underserved populations, and the assurance that hepatitis prevention and treatment efforts are patient-centered, and connect to necessary behavioral health, drug treatment, and social services.[45] The 2024 budget proposed by the White House sets aside $12.3 billion over the next 10 years to eliminate HCV through the expansion of testing, increased access to DAAs, and decreased cost of curative treatments. The proposed plan has 4 key components.

- Identify more cases by expanding access to single-visit, rapid results testing
- Expand access to care by eliminating burdensome requirements for people using Medicaid
- Lower costs by establishing a subscription model wherein the government negotiates lump sum medications (aka, "Netflix" model)
- Invest in community health programs that are best suited to deliver care while also working to develop a hepatitis C vaccine

This program would focus on populations with high infection levels while bolstering provider capacity and public health efforts to enhance communication and surveillance.[46]

SUMMARY

Immense progress has been made since the discovery of HCV in 1989 followed by the development of curative therapies that eradicate infection over 95% of the time. The safety, high efficacy, and simplicity of HCV antiviral regimens provide a rare opportunity to eliminate a worldwide, life-threatening viral infection. DAAs bolster the opportunity to reduce the HCV viral burden on a population-based level through large-scale treatment as prevention programs if there's a well-integrated care delivery model to reach those most impacted by the disease. Several structural barriers and gaps in the HCV care continuum pose challenges to this goal. With the first US National Hepatitis C Elimination Initiative pending Congressional fund allocation, there is an opportunity to mobilize to combat the growing burden of HCV in ways that breakdown stigma, social, and institutional barriers to care. With increased public awareness, widespread advocacy and the provision of low-threshold social, and clinical services to marginalized groups, the United States can make additional strides to advance elimination goals to reach international and national benchmarks. The pharmaceutical tools to facilitate widespread treatment uptake and resultant cure are readily available, but the foundational infrastructure to reach more people requires fiscal backing with well-planned public health organization and investment. With joined forces, HCV elimination is achievable and could mark a modern-day medical miracle.

CLINICS CARE POINTS

- Every adult should be tested for HCV Ab.
- If there are ongoing risk factors for HCV exposure, repeat HCV screening is indicated.
- Once an HCV Ab test results positive, an HCV RNA is needed to confirm active infection.
- Once diagnosed, HCV treatment should not be deferred.
- Direct-acting antivirals require daily adherence for 8-12 weeks with minimal side effects. Once cured, the HCV Ab remains positive lifelong and will not protect against reinfection.

REFERENCES

1. Hofmeister MG, Rosenthal EM, Barker LK, et al. Estimating prevalence of hepatitis C virus infection in the United States, 2013-2016. Hepatology 2019;69(3): 1020–31.
2. Thompson WW, Symum H, Sandul A, et al. *Vital signs:* hepatitis C treatment among insured adults — United States, 2019–2020. MMWR Morb Mortal Wkly Rep 2022;71:1011–7.
3. Dhiman RK, Premkumar M. Hepatitis C virus elimination by 2030: conquering mount improbable. Clin Liver Dis 2021;16(6):254–61.
4. Yehia BR, Schranz AJ, Umscheid CA, et al. 3rd. The treatment cascade for chronic hepatitis C virus infection in the United States: a systematic review and meta-analysis. PLoS One 2014;9(7).
5. Holmberg SD, Spradling PR, Moorman AC, et al. Hepatitis C in the United States. N Engl J Med 2013;368(20):1859–61.
6. Denniston MM, Klevens RM, McQuillan GM, et al. Awareness of infection, knowledge of hepatitis C, and medical follow-up among individuals testing positive for hepatitis C: national Health and Nutrition Examination Survey 2001-2008. Hepatology 2012;55(6):1652–61.
7. Kim HS, Yang JD, El-Serag HB, et al. Awareness of chronic viral hepatitis in the United States: an update from the national health and nutrition examination Survey. J Viral Hepat 2019;26(5):596–602.
8. Centers for Disease Control and Prevention. Viral hepatitis surveillance report – United States. 2021. Available at: https://www.cdc.gov/hepatitis/statistics/2021surveillance/index.htm.2023. Accessed October 1, 2024.
9. Klevens RM, Liu S, Roberts H, et al. Estimating acute viral hepatitis infections from nationally reported cases. Am J Publ Health 2014;104:482–7.
10. Edlin BR, Eckhardt BJ, Shu MA, et al. Toward a more accurate estimate of the prevalence of hepatitis C in the United States. Hepatology 2015;62(5):1353–63.
11. Hall EW, Bradley H, Barker LK, et al. Estimating hepatitis C prevalence in the United States, 2017–2020. Hepatology 2024;10:1097.
12. Collier MF, Holtzman D, Holmberg SD. Hepatitis C virus. In: Long SS, Prober CG, Fisher M, editors. Principles and practice of pediatric infectious diseases. 5th edition. Philadelphia, PA: Elsevier; 2018. p. 1135–41.

13. Westbrook RH, Dusheiko G. Natural history of hepatitis C. J Hepatol 2014; 61(Suppl 1):S58–68.

14. Ly KN, Miniño AM, Liu SJ, et al. Deaths associated with hepatitis C virus infection among residents in 50 states and the District of Columbia, 2016-2017. Clin Infect Dis 2020;71(5):1149–60.

15. Schillie SF, Canary L, Koneru A, et al. Hepatitis C virus in women of childbearing age, pregnant women, and children. Am J Prev Med 2018;55:633–41.

16. Pakianathan M, Whittaker W, Lee M, et al. Chemsex and new HIV diagnosis in gay, bisexual and other men who have sex with men attending sexual health clinics. HIV Med 2018;19(7):485–90.

17. AASLD and IDSA. HCV guidance: recommendations for testing, managing, and treating hepatitis C. 2024. Available at: www.hcvguidelines.org. Accessed October 1, 2024.

18. Nwaohiri A, Schillie S, Bulterys M, et al. Towards elimination of hepatitis C virus infection in children. Lancet Child Adolesc Health 2018;2:235–7.

19. Nwaohiri A, Schillie S, Bulterys M, et al. Hepatitis C virus infection in children: how do we prevent it and how do we treat it? Expert Rev Anti Infect Ther 2018;16: 689–94.

20. Benova L, Mohamoud YA, Calvert C, et al. Vertical transmission of hepatitis C virus: systematic review and meta-analysis. Clin Infect Dis 2014;59:765–73.

21. Schillie S, Wester C, Osborne M, et al. CDC recommendations for hepatitis C screening among adults - United States, 2020. MMWR Recomm Rep (Morb Mortal Wkly Rep) 2020;69(2):1–17.

22. Panagiotakopoulos L, Sandul AL, DHSc, et al. CDC recommendations for hepatitis C testing among perinatally exposed infants and children — United States, 2023. MMWR Recomm Rep (Morb Mortal Wkly Rep) 2023;72(RR-4):1–19.

23. Blanding DP, Moran WP, Bian J, et al. Linkage to specialty care in the hepatitis C care cascade. J Invest Med 2021;69(2):324–32.

24. Falade-Nwulia O, Kim N. Addressing structural barriers to HCV treatment. In: Hepatitis C online. 2024. Available at: https://www.hepatitisc.uw.edu/go/evaluation-treatment/addressing-structural-barriers-to-treatment/core-concept/all. Accessed October 1, 2024.

25. Talal AH, Markatou M, Liu A, et al. Integrated hepatitis c-opioid use disorder care through facilitated telemedicine: a randomized trial. JAMA 2024;331(16):1369.

26. Marcellin P, Boyer N, Gervais A, et al. Long-term histologic improvement and loss of detectable intrahepatic HCV RNA in patients with chronic hepatitis C and sustained response to interferon-alpha therapy. Ann Intern Med 1997;127(10): 875–81.

27. Centers for Disease Control and Prevention (CDC). Testing for HCV infection: an update of guidance for clinicians and laboratorians. MMWR Morb Mortal Wkly Rep 2013;62(18):362–5.

28. Spach D. Initial evaluation of persons with chronic HCV. In: Hepatitis C online. 2024. Available at: https://www.hepatitisc.uw.edu/go/evaluation-staging-monitoring/initial-evaluation-chronic/core-concept/all#general-approach-to-initial-evaluation. Accessed October 1, 2024.

29. Chou R, Wasson N. Blood tests to diagnose fibrosis or cirrhosis in patients with chronic hepatitis C virus infection: a systematic review. Ann Intern Med 2013; 158(11):807–20.

30. Feld JJ, Jacobson IM, Hézode C, et al, ASTRAL-1 Investigators. Sofosbuvir and velpatasvir for HCV genotype 1, 2, 4, 5, and 6 infection. N Engl J Med 2015; 373(27):2599.

31. Mangia A, Milligan S, Khalili M, et al. Global real-world evidence of sofosbuvir/velpatasvir as simple, effective HCV treatment: analysis of 5552 patients from 12 cohorts. Liver Int 2020;40(8):1841–52.
32. Dufour JF, Zuckerman E, Zadeikis N, et al. Safety of glecaprevir/pibrentasvir in adults with chronic genotype 1-6 hepatitis C virus infection: an integrated analysis. Amsterdam, The Netherlands: Presented at the 52nd Annual Meeting of the European Association for the Study of the Liver (EASL); 2017.
33. Zeuzem S, Foster GR, Wang S, et al. Glecaprevir-pibrentasvir for 8 or 12 Weeks in HCV genotype 1 or 3 infection. N Engl J Med 2018;378(4):354–69.
34. Lampertico P, Carrión JA, Curry M, et al. Real-world effectiveness and safety of glecaprevir/pibrentasvir for the treatment of patients with chronic HCV infection: a meta-analysis. J Hepatol 2020;72(6):1112–21.
35. Brzdęk M, Zarębska-Michaluk D, Invernizzi F, et al. Decade of optimizing therapy with direct-acting antiviral drugs and the changing profile of patients with chronic hepatitis C. World J Gastroenterol 2023;29(6):949–66.
36. Rong L, Perelson AS. Treatment of hepatitis C virus infection with interferon and small molecule direct antivirals: viral kinetics and modeling. Crit Rev Immunol 2010;30(2):131–48.
37. HepVu. Hepatitis C treatment restrictions. In: HepVu. 2022. Available at: https://hepvu.org/news-updates/hepatitis-c-treatment-restrictions-2/. Accessed October 1, 2024.
38. Arora S, Thornton K, Murata G, et al. Outcomes of treatment for hepatitis C virus infection by primary care providers. N Engl J Med 2011;364(23):2199–207.
39. Irvin R, Ntiri-Reid B, Kleinman M, et al. Sharing the cure: building primary care and public health infrastructure to improve the hepatitis C care continuum in Maryland. J Viral Hepat 2020;27(12):1388–95.
40. Arora S, Thornton K, Jenkusky SM, et al. Project ECHO: linking university specialists with rural and prison-based clinicians to improve care for people with chronic hepatitis C in New Mexico. Publ Health Rep 2007;122(Suppl 2):74–7.
41. University of California, San Francisco. National clinician consultation center. Available at: https://nccc.ucsf.edu/clinician-consultation/hepatitis-c-management/. Accessed October 1, 2024.
42. World Health Organization. Treatment of adolescents and children with chronic HCV infection, and HCV simplified service delivery and diagnostics. 2022. Available at: https://www.who.int/publications/i/item/9789240052734.
43. World Health Organization. Guidelines for the care and treatment of persons diagnosed with chronic hepatitis C infection. 2018. Available at: https://www.who.int/publications/i/item/9789241550345. Accessed October 1, 2024.
44. Centers for Disease Control and Prevention. Division of viral hepatitis 2025 strategic plan. Available at: https://www.cdc.gov/hepatitis/media/DVH-StrategicPlan2020-2025. Accessed October 1, 2024.
45. Valdiserri RO, Koh HK, Ward J. Overcome health inequities to eliminate viral hepatitis. JAMA 2023;329(19):1637–8.
46. Coalition for global hepatitis elimination/the Task force for global health. US National Hepatitis C Elimination Initiative 2024. Available at: https://www.globalhep.org/advocacy/united-states-national-hepatitis-c-elimination-initiative. Accessed October 1, 2024.
47. Bourne A, Reid D, Hickson F, et al. Illicit drug use in sexual settings ('chemsex') and HIV/STI transmission risk behaviour among gay men in South London: findings from a qualitative study. Sex Transm Infect 2015;91(8):564–8.

Syphilis Update

Daniel P. Worrall, MSN, ANP-BC

KEYWORDS

- Sexually transmitted disease • Syphilis • *T pallidum* • Men who have sex with men
- Public health nursing • Sexual health

KEY POINTS

- Although men who have sex with men continue to be adversely affected, record rates of infection are now seen in women, men who have sex with women, and in congenital cases.
- Stages of the infection are marked by an array of symptoms that can easily be confused with other diseases or conditions.
- Two testing algorithms are used to identify new infection and follow patients to ensure cure.
- Penicillin remains the recommended treatment in all stages.
- Careful review of sexual and social history is key to identifying patients at risk and those presenting with symptoms.

INTRODUCTION

As a clinician, there is nothing more worrisome than a missed or misdiagnosis. The patient presenting with nonspecific symptoms can spark anxiety among nurses who triage. Fever, swollen glands, headache, myalgias, rash? The differential diagnosis can be pages long. Now imagine that diagnosis is elusive, the last thing on your radar, an infection most believe is a thing of the past: syphilis. Rates in the United States have reached record highs and continue to climb annually. Until recently, the infection disproportionately affected gender and minority populations but is rapidly expanding to include other groups. Now, more than ever it is important to recognize symptoms and those at risk.

THE GREAT IMITATOR

Syphilis is a systemic infection caused by the bacteria *Treponema pallidum*, a spirochete usually transmitted through oral, vaginal, or anal sex, but also congenitally from mother to unborn baby. In sexual transmission, the bacteria enter through a microabrasion or microtrauma to the mucosa where it rapidly multiplies before moving to the lymphatics where it is then quickly disseminated throughout the body.[1–3] Unlike other

Massachusetts General Hospital, Sexual Health Clinic, 55 Fruit Street, Cox Building, 5th Floor, Boston, MA 02114, USA
E-mail address: dworrall@mgh.harvard.edu

Nurs Clin N Am 60 (2025) 523–535
https://doi.org/10.1016/j.cnur.2024.10.001
0029-6465/25/© 2024 Elsevier Inc. All rights reserved, including those for text and data mining, AI training, and similar technologies.

bacterial infections, the organism evades the immune system making clearance impossible without treatment. Syphilis presents in 3 stages—each manifesting different symptoms that are easily confused with other diseases or infections (**Table 1**).

Primary Syphilis

The first stage is marked by the development of a "chancre" at the site of infection. (**Figs. 1** and **2**) Chancres first appear as a papule that quickly erodes into a nonexudative ulcer with heaped, indurated edges. Symptoms can appear anywhere from 1 week to 3 months after transmission but in most cases manifest around 3 weeks.[2,3] Chancres are teeming with spirochetes and highly infectious. Local lymph adenopathy is usually present. Despite being regarded as painless in most cases, the chancre may be tender or irritating depending on where it is located and what it comes in contact with (ie, urine, clothing). Atypical presentations are common in patients with human immunodeficiency virus (HIV) and may include more than one ulcer.[2,3] Without treatment, chancres will heal. Patients may rationalize away what may have caused it in the first place and not seek care. "I must have cut myself shaving." "I think I caught myself in my zipper." Those who do seek care will likely undergo work-up for other ulcerative diseases like herpes. Chancres are likely to go unnoticed if located inside the vagina or rectum.

Secondary Syphilis

Untreated patients will enter the second stage of infection marked by the development of a maculopapular rash (**Figs. 3** and **4**). This occurs within 2 to 24 weeks after transmission, either as the chancre is resolving or shortly following.[2,3] The presentation we are taught to look for is an erythematous macular rash on the palms of the hands or soles of the feet, but more often this will appear on the trunk, back, or extremities. It may also present as annular, pustular, or have scale.[4] It is most often not itchy despite its appearance. Patients often notice this getting out of the shower as it tends to darken when wet. As a nurse, you will be searching for potential allergens or asking about insect bites or new medications. You may go down the fungal dermatitis route. Patients in this stage may report being febrile, having pharyngitis, new-onset myalgias/arthralgias, or patchy, unexplained hair loss. These symptoms are generic

Table 1
Infectious syphilis staging and symptoms

Primary (1 wk 3 mo After Infection)	Secondary (2–24 wk After Infection)	Latent/Late Infection
• Chancre develops at the site of infection—usually painless ulcer with heaped, indurated edges. May be in the mouth, on the penis, vagina, or inside the rectum • Local lymph adenopathy-cervical, inguinal	• Maculopapular rash develops just before or shortly following resolution of chancre. Does not typically itch, may be on the palms or soles of the feet but also the back, trunk, and extremities • Fever • Myalgias/arthralgias • Pharyngitis • Patch hair loss • Condyloma lata (rapidly growing anogenital warts)	• No appreciable signs or symptoms • Patients remain infectious for up to 1 yr • If untreated, patients will eventually enter the tertiary stage where symptoms of neurologic, cardiovascular, and gummatous lesions manifest

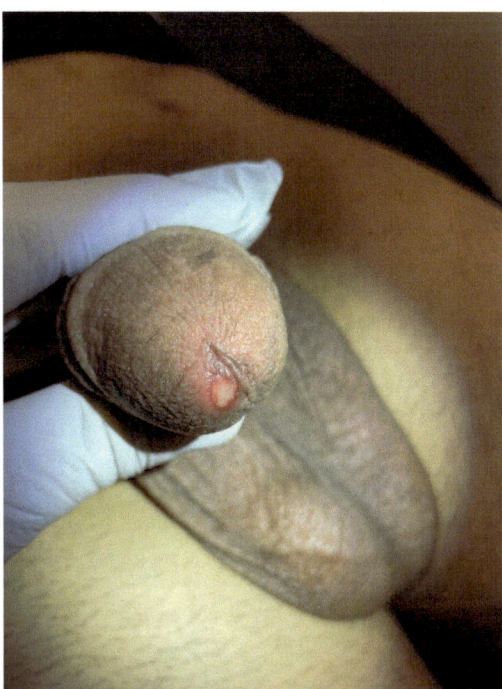

Fig. 1. Penile chancre – primary syphilis (*Image courtesy of* D. Worrall, NP, 2024, reprinted with permission.)

enough to warrant extensive work-up by clinicians. Rapidly growing anogenital warts known as condyloma lata, or mucus patches in the mouth or on the labia in women or prepuce in men, are other manifestations of secondary syphilis, often triggering another diagnosis or work-up. Without treatment, the rash and other symptoms will eventually resolve. Both clinician and patient will be left scratching their heads.

Latent and Congenital Infection

Syphilis persisting beyond primary and secondary stages is the most elusive of all. After a year, patients are no longer infectious and no longer presenting with symptoms.[2,3] Decades will go by where the organism *T pallidum* will continue to evade the immune system. Unless the infection is picked up on serology testing, the patient will eventually enter a tertiary stage of disease. Patients will suffer damage to vessels, bones, and soft tissues, including vital organs like the heart, liver, and brain. Fibrous, granulomatous masses called gummas will form throughout the body. In this late stage, the diagnosis is often made via rule-out testing when someone suffers a seizure or undergoes work-up for a cardiac arrhythmia.

Syphilis spread congenitally from mother to unborn baby results in devastating consequences including prematurity, low birth weight, skeletal abnormalities, developmental delay, neonatal death, or loss of the pregnancy.[5,6] Routine testing has been implemented to detect these cases, though delays can be seen in marginalized populations with little access to or who do not seek care. It is imperative that all patients of childbearing potential at risk be tested to detect infection early. As treatment can have adverse effects on the pregnancy, these cases are usually treated in a monitored setting under close supervision.

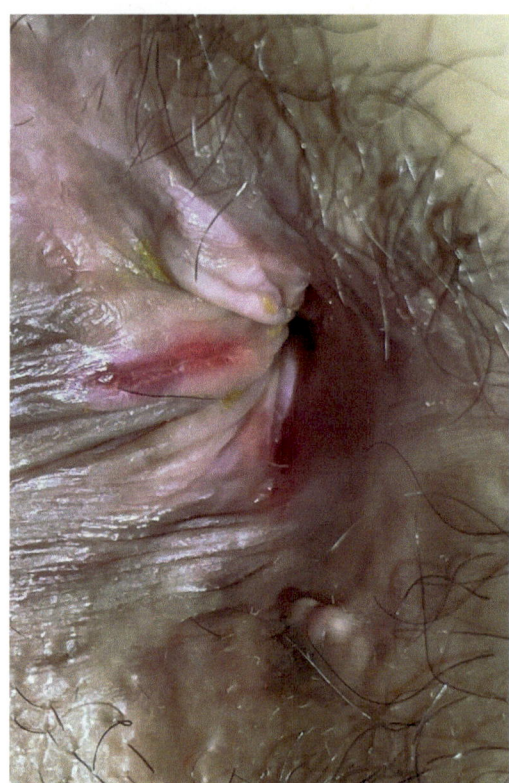

Fig. 2. Anal chancre – primary syphilis (*Image courtesy of* D. Worrall, NP, 2023, reprinted with permission.)

BACK WITH A VENGEANCE

Infectious syphilis in the United States reached an all-time low in the year 2000, with only 5,979 cases of primary and secondary infection.[7] The latest surveillance data released by the Centers for Disease Control and Prevention (CDC) in 2023 revealed that 209,253 new cases were reported. This is the greatest number since 1950, a 61.1% increase over the previous 5 years. Despite an increase of only 1% from 2022, rates of reported cases in the population remain stable. Variations are seen in different groups. So who is being infected?

Since the rise in cases in 2001, Men who have sex with men (MSM) have been disproportionately impacted. From 2014 to 2023 MSM represented the largest percentage of primary and secondary cases at 44.9%. In 2023, they accounted for 32.7% of these cases, 17,331, a decrease of 13.4% from the year prior, the first substantial decrease in the last 15 years.[7] Infections have rapidly spread to other groups. Despite modest decreases in primary and secondary cases in the last year in women and men who have sex with women (MSW), overall infections remain high. There were 13,763 cases of primary and secondary syphilis reported among women in 2023, a 6.1% decrease from 2022. In MSW there were 12,829 of these cases reported in 2023, a 4.0% decrease from the year prior. What is most significant is a look at the last 5 years. This reveals how widespread syphilis has become in the general population and how narrow the difference is between genders and their sexual practices. (**Fig. 5**). From 2019 to 2023, the number of cases in MSM decreased 5.7%, while

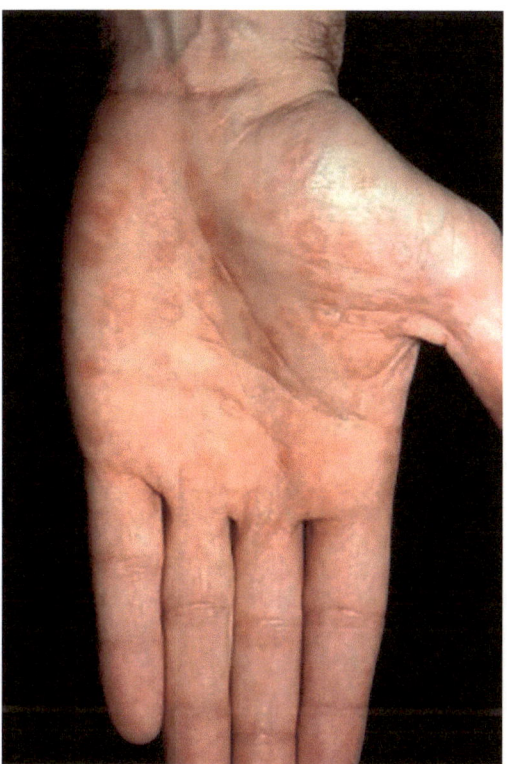

Fig. 3. Palmar macules—secondary syphilis. (William D. James, Dirk M. Elston, James R. Treat, Misha A. Rosenbach. Andrews' Diseases of the Skin: Clinical Dermatology, 14 Edition, Elsevier Inc, 2024.)

the number of cases increased 112.0% in women, and 76.0% in MSW. Men who have sex with unknown (MSU), where the gender of sexual partners is unknown, saw a 34.1% increase in cases.

Ethnic minorities have seen persistent increases in infection rates, with a surprisingly sharp increase in non-Hispanic American Indian or Alaska Natives since 2020,

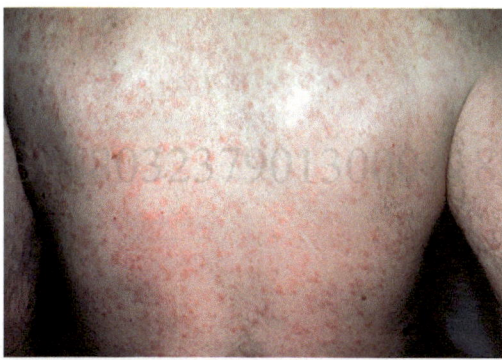

Fig. 4. Secondary syphilis. (Robert G. Micheletti, William D. James, Dirk M. Elston, Patrick J. McMahon, Andrews' Diseases of the Skin Clinical Atlas. 2nd Edition, 2021, Elsevier.)

Primary and Secondary Syphilis — Reported Cases by Sex and Sex of Sex Partners and Year, United States, 2014–2023

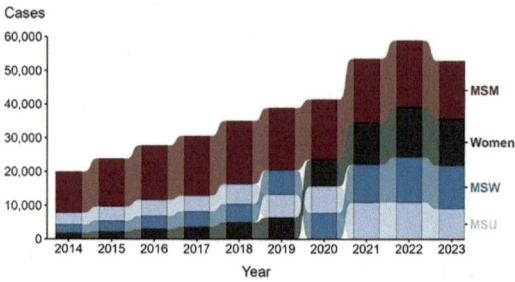

Fig. 5. Primary and secondary syphilis cases by sex and sex of partners. MSM, men who have sex with men; MSW, men who have sex with women only; MSU, men who have sex with partners of unknown gender. (From CDC Syphilis Slides from STI Surveillance, 2023.)

followed by a steady rise in non-Hispanic Black/African Americas and persons of multiracial background.[8] Whites and Hispanic/Latinos rates have seen a more gradual trend (**Fig. 6**).

Substance use and certain sexual behaviors have helped fuel syphilis cases in recent years. In 2022, 11.8% of all primary and secondary cases were in someone reporting methamphetamine use, 7.0% reported injection drug use, 3.8% reported cocaine use, 2.2% heroin use, and 1.5% crack use.[8] Nearly all types of substance use have seen increases over the 5 years, with the most significant in methamphetamine use (**Fig. 7**). Sex with anonymous partners was reported in 59.7% of all primary and secondary syphilis cases involving MSM, 38.7% in MSW, and 20.1% in women. Sex with an active substance user, sex in exchange for money or something of need, recent incarceration, and unstable housing or homelessness were additional circumstances preceding infection across the population.[8]

Perhaps the most disturbing trend is seen in congenital syphilis. In 2023, there were a total of 3,882 cases reported in the United States, including 279 congenital-related stillbirths and neonatal/infant deaths. This is an increase of 3.0% from the year prior, and is the largest number of congenital syphilis cases since 1992. From 2019 to 2023 there has been a 104.4% increase women diagnosed with syphilis during their pregnancy.[5,7] Cases are directly related to the ongoing rise in cases of primary and

Primary and Secondary Syphilis — Rates of Reported Cases by Race/Hispanic Ethnicity and Year, United States, 2019–2023

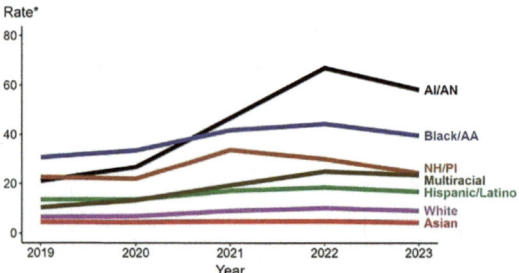

Fig. 6. Primary and secondary syphilis by race and ethnicity. [a]Per 100,000. AI/AN, American Indian or Alaskan native; Black/AA, Black or African American; NH/PI, native Hawaiian or other Pacific Islander. (From CDC Syphilis Slides from STI Surveillance, 2023.)

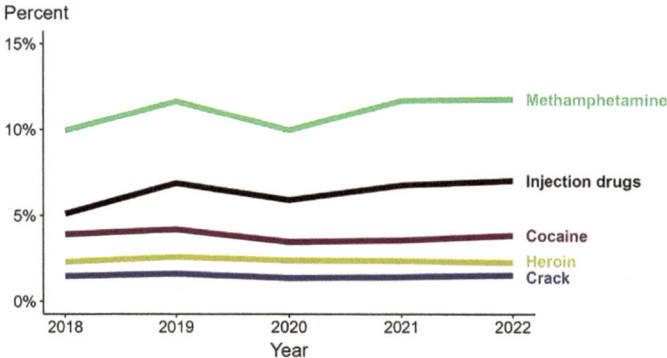

Fig. 7. Primary and secondary syphilis by substance use behaviors. [a]Proportion reporting injection drug use, methamphetamine use, heroin use, crack use, or cocaine use within the last 12 months calculated among cases with known data (cases with missing or unknown responses were excluded from the denominator). (*From* CDC Syphilis Surveillance Supplemental Slides 2018-2022.)

secondary syphilis in women of reproductive age. Maternal risk factors for syphilis during pregnancy include sex with multiple partners, sex in conjunction with drug use or transactional sex, late entry to prenatal care or no prenatal care, methamphetamine or heroin use, incarceration of the woman or her partner, and unstable housing or homelessness.[5,6]

IDENTIFYING INFECTIONS

Nurses are on the frontlines of public health and are often the first to interact with patients in crisis or triage patients with concerning symptoms or questions. According to a recent Gallup Poll, nurses continue to be rated America's most trusted profession for their honesty and ethical standards.[9] In addition to symptomatology, history taking is an essential step in identifying patients at risk and getting them into care. With sexual practices and substance use being a highly sensitive, private aspect of a patient's life, trust is essential to opening dialogue. It is a privilege to be invited into this realm that with it carries heavy responsibility. We all have our own styles, but there are several important points to remember.

Start by making sure that the clinical space supports the patient. This should be welcoming of all gender identities, sexual orientations, races, and ethnicities. Privacy and confidentiality should be reinforced. Patients should always be seen without partners, friends, or family so they may be comfortable discussing aspects of their lives they may not choose to share with others. There may also be a history of trauma or domestic violence to consider. Remind patients that sexual health is part of general health. Reassure patients that substance use and other behaviors are common and what they disclose is kept confidential. Use plain, matter-of-fact language and keep your poker face. Nothing should be shocking or warrant a negative reaction.

When taking a sexual history, the CDC recommends using the 5 "P"s: *Partners, Practices, Protection* from sexually transmitted infections (STIs), *Past* History of STIs, and *Pregnancy* Intention.[10] These are meant to provide framework for a discussion but it is hardly one-size-fits-all. Each patient and situation is unique and interviewing should be tailored accordingly.

Partners

Information on partners includes gender and gender identity of partners and the number of these partners in a given timeframe. Do you have sex with men, women, transgendered men or women, nonbinary, or people of other gender identity? How many partners have you had sexual contact within the last week? Month? Year? Do you have a steady/regular partner? Are you in a relationship? Is it monogamous, or open? Do you have partners outside the relationship? Do you ever engage in sex with more than one partner, or group sex?

Practices

It is important not to assume sexual practices when working with patients of any gender identity, sexual orientation, or age. Use clear, plain language to identify potential exposures. Explain to the patient that it is important to know where we need to test for infections. Expand on the question "When was the last time you had sexual contact?" to include specific activities. When was the last time you gave or received oral sex? Has someone else's penis been in or around your anus? If so, when? Has anyone had their mouth on your anus, or have you had your mouth on someone else's? When was the last time you had vaginal or anal sex or inserted your penis into someone's vagina or anus? When appropriate, use vernacular specific to how the patient may identify. When was the last time you bottomed (received anal sex/had a penis inside the anus)? When was the last time you topped (penis inside someone else's anus)? Do you ever rim or get rimmed (oral-anal contact)?

Protection

Protection is unfortunately in the eye of the beholder. Some patients may see protection as contraception or may qualify certain activities where they feel they need to be protected. It is important to be specific. When you last had vaginal or anal sex, did you use a condom? How frequently do use condoms in general—sometimes, always, never? What prevents you from using condoms? Do you use barriers for oral sex? In the age of HIV pre-exposure prophylaxis (PrEP) and doxycycline post-exposure prophylaxis (doxy PEP), it is important to ask about these and introduce them to patients who may be appropriate. Have you heard of HIV PrEP? For patients who are already taking ask about adherence. How often do you miss a dose? Has anyone ever talked to you about doxy PEP, or doxy PEP?

Past Infection

It is important to know about a patient's history of STIs, both as a risk factor for getting other STIs, but also to identify patients with a past infection of syphilis. This becomes important in following patients after treatment. Have you ever had gonorrhea, chlamydia, or syphilis in the past? When was the last time? Were you treated? Was your partner treated? Was gonorrhea in your throat, penis, or anus? Did you have follow-up testing to make sure it was gone? Patients reporting recurrent infections are at high risk for HIV and other complications. They should be offered HIV PrEP and doxy PEP as part of care.

Pregnancy

Finally, given the record rates of congenital syphilis, asking about pregnancy is essential. Are you on a form of birth control/contraception? When was your last menstrual cycle? Is there a chance you could be pregnant?

Ask about other activities related to sex and encourage questions. Do you use any substances when you have sex, like poppers, crystal methamphetamine, cocaine, marijuana? How often do you have sex while under the influence of alcohol or other substances? Have you ever experienced domestic violence or sexual assault? Do you have any questions or concerns about sex? Do you have any questions about STIs or what you can do to protect yourself? Make sure to ask whether they are a known contact to an STI. Has anyone contacted you to tell you they had an infection like gonorrhea, chlamydia, or syphilis?

TESTING, TREATMENT, AND FOLLOW-UP

Obtaining a good history and identifying symptoms will guide testing. Ask about ulcers or sores on the mouth, penis, vulva, or anus. Ask if the patient experiences any pain with sex. Inquire about fever, sore throat, swollen glands in the neck or groin. Ask about rash. Patients who present with symptoms suspicious of syphilis should be tested and treated per guidelines. Aside from dark field microscopy where a specialized illumination technique is used to identify spirochetes, serology is the only way to test for syphilis. Patients under high suspicion should be treated presumptively while awaiting confirmation as long as treatment is available. Confirmed infections must be reported to the Department of Public Health in all 50 states for both public health efforts and to assist in partner notification and treatment when necessary.

Testing

The CDC recommends 2 algorithms based on clinical resources[11] (**Fig. 8**). In the traditional algorithm, a non-treponemal test like the rapid plasma reagin (RPR) or venereal disease research laboratory test looks for antibodies that react to lipoidal antigens present in syphilis and other inflammatory conditions. The most common used in the

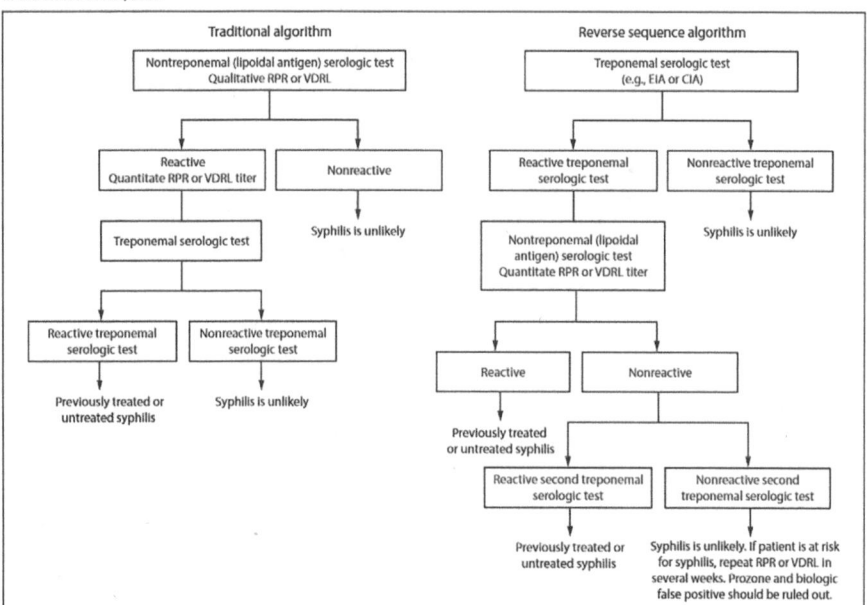

Fig. 8. CDC laboratory recommendations for syphilis testing. CIA, chemiluminescence immunoassay; EIA, enzyme immunoassay; RPR, rapid plasma regain; TPPA, *Treponema pallidum* particle agglutination; VDRL, venereal disease research laboratory. (*From* CDC Laboratory Recommendations for Syphilis Testing, United States, 2024.)

United States is the RPR. When positive, a titer is calculated based on reactivity in the sample and increased exponentially—that is, nonreactive (NR), 1:1, 1:2, 1:4, 1:8, and so forth. Titers can rise to over 1,000 in primary and secondary stages of infection. As this test can be positive in other inflammatory conditions, pregnancy, IV drug use, and old age, a treponemal-specific test is needed to confirm the presence of *T pallidum*.

The reverse algorithm starts with a treponemal-specific test and reflexes to the nonspecific RPR. A florescent treponemal antibody test (FTA-ABS), *T pallidum* particle agglutination assay (TP-PA), and syphilis enzyme-linked immunoassays are commonly used, and more recently chemiluminescence immunoassay and multiplex flow (microbead) immunoassays. These identify antibodies specific to *T pallidum* and will usually stay positive for an infected person's lifetime. An RPR will be performed to stage the infection. Titers climb during primary syphilis, peak during secondary syphilis, and decline as patients enter latent infection (even without treatment). Most settings where testing is frequent operate on the reverse algorithm, identifying presence of the organism that causes syphilis before running the nonspecific RPR.

Ordering tests and reading results can be confusing for clinicians. It is important to remember that antibodies specific to *T pallidum* will usually remain positive throughout a patient's life. Therefore, treponemal-specific tests cannot be used to identify reinfection and are not useful in patients with a history of syphilis. Similarly, nonspecific tests cannot be used alone to confirm a diagnosis of syphilis. RPRs are the key in management, however. The RPR is not only used to stage the infection but also followed for some time after treatment to ensure cure. Titers return to nonreactive. Some individuals may be *serofast*, which is when there is a low titer (usually 1:1 or 1:2) that persists following effective treatment and clearance of the infection. Individuals who are serofast are not infectious.

Treatment

In the age of antibiotic resistance, it is amazing that syphilis continues to be sensitive to penicillin in all stages of the disease (**Table 2**). In primary, secondary, and latent infection, long-acting penicillin G is administered by deep intramuscular (IM) injection. The usual treatment dose is 2.4 million units.[12,13] Patients with primary, secondary, and early latent infection (infection sometime within the previous 12 months) are treated with a single dose. Infections of unknown duration, or late latent syphilis, are given this dose weekly for 3 weeks. Patients should see full resolution of symptoms with treatment. In tertiary stages, intravenous (IV) administration may be necessary for

Table 2
Recommended treatment of syphilis

Primary and secondary syphilis	Benzathine penicillin G 2.4 million units IM in a single dose
Early Latent Syphilis (infection of <12 mo)	Benzathine penicillin G 2.4 million units IM in a single dose
Late Latent Syphilis (infection >12 mo, or of unknown duration without neurologic involvement)	Benzathine penicillin G 7.2 million units total, administered as 3 doses of 2.4 million units IM each at 1 wk intervals
Tertiary Syphilis without Neurologic Involvement	Benzathine penicillin G 7.2 million units total, administered as 3 doses of 2.4 million units IM each at 1 wk intervals
Neurosyphilis, Ocular Syphilis, Otosyphilis, Congenital Syphilis	Aqueous crystalline penicillin G

Box 1
Populations at risk for infection

- Men who have sex with men (MSM)
- Persons in higher risk communities including American Indian/Alaskan Natives and African Americans
- All persons using substances during or at the time of sexual contact
- Persons who exchange sex for money or something they need
- Persons suffering from unstable housing or homelessness
- Persons with recent incarceration

---

involvement of the eyes, brain, or other organs and patients can expect sequelae from advanced disease. Suspected or congenital cases have extensive work-up and are treated with a combination of both IM and IV administration.

Alternatives to penicillin are few. Depending on the stage and patient, persons with penicillin allergy could be offered a course of doxycycline, dosed 100 mg twice a day for 2 to 4 weeks.[12] As one can imagine, side effects, tolerability, and adherence are real issues with this treatment. Desensitization to penicillin is recommended in pregnancy and in high-risk cases such as those with late-stage infection.

Patients who are treated for primary and secondary infection should be informed of the potential for a Jarisch-Herxheimer reaction. This is an acute, immune-mediated process within the first 24 hours of receiving penicillin where patients may experience fever, headache, or myalgia.[2,12] This can be treated with over-the-counter analgesics and antipyretics and reassurance from providers. This is most commonly seen in patients with secondary syphilis presumably due to bacterial load. Patients should be instructed to notify all sexual partners in the last 3 months so they may be tested and treated as contacts. Patient must refrain from *all* sexual activities for 7 days after treatment or for 7 days after all sexual contacts have been treated. Patients treated for latent syphilis requiring treatment administered several weeks should be made aware that the dosing schedule must not deviate beyond a day or the treatment course will need to be repeated. All patients should be educated that syphilis is bacteria and they can be reinfected in the future.

As with any other sexually transmitted infection, patients with syphilis should be tested for HIV. Patients with ulcerative disease are at higher risk for HIV transmission.[2,14] According to the CDC, 36% of MSM diagnosed with primary and secondary syphilis in 2022 were HIV positive, increasing the risk of coinfection among their partners.[8] PrEP and doxy PEP should be offered to MSM and other patients where appropriate. Recent study has shown that doxy PEP could reduce transmission of syphilis

---

Box 2
The 5 "P"s of sexual history taking

Partners

Practices

Protection from STIs

Past History of STIs

Pregnancy Intention

Adapted from CDC Guide to Sexual History Taking.

---

by up to 70% in MSM and transgender women.[15] This may be responsible for the recent decline in cases in MSM.

Follow-up

It is vital that patients treated for syphilis have follow-up. Clinical manifestations should resolve with treatment, and a decline should be seen in RPR from baseline. The CDC recommends all patients treated for syphilis have follow-up serologies at 6, 12, and 24 months after treatment.[12] Clinicians may decide to repeat these earlier to keep patients engaged in care. Failure of patients to achieve a fourfold decrease in RPR within 24 months after treatment may mean reinfection or treatment failure and patients should be considered for retreatment. Titers less than 1:8 are not as likely to decline as rapidly as those that are elevated.

SUMMARY

To say that syphilis is becoming a public health crisis in the United States is an understatement. Although MSM continue to be adversely affected by the disease, women and MSW are seeing record rates of infection. Substance use, sexual behaviors, and other social circumstances like unstable housing or incarceration influence the likelihood of being infected. The congenital rate in the United States is unacceptable. Pregnant women at risk for infection must be tested and treated appropriately to avoid serious complications, fetal injury, or death. Identifying populations at risk is imperative to getting ahead of this epidemic (**Box 1**). Knowing what symptoms to look for in patients and what to ask is vital. History taking is a skill that will guide testing (**Box 2**). Knowing what tests to order and how to interpret results will soon become second nature. These patients need prompt treatment and longitudinal follow-up to ensure cure. As nurses, we have always been those who educate and inform. Starting the conversation about sexual health and making patients feel comfortable is key to invoking change. Provide information on protection that goes beyond condoms to include PrEP or doxy PEP in patients at risk. It is important to encourage routine STI screening as part of general health. Syphilis may be back with a vengeance, but it has met its match with the nursing community. We can identify, treat, educate, and help prevent the spread of infection.

CLINICS CARE POINTS

- Always educate patients regarding transmission and the potential for reinfection.
- Suspected cases should be treated while awaiting test results to avoid morbidity and further transmission.
- Patients of childbearing potential who have syphilis *must* be tested for pregnancy and referred for treatment in a monitored setting.
- Advise patients to refrain from *all* sexual contact for 7 days after treatment, and for 7 days after all partners have been treated.
- All sexual partners of the previous 3 months should be evaluated and treated as contacts of those infected regardless of symptoms. Engage your local department of public health for anonymous partner notification when needed.
- Remind patients that they may experience a Jarisch-Herxheimer reaction following treatment where they may feel febrile or have muscle or joint aches. This can be treated with over-the-counter remedies and provider reassurance.
- Follow patients for symptom resolution. An RPR should be drawn at 6 and 12 months to check for 4 fold drop in titer to ensure cure. Testing may be done sooner to keep patients engaged in care.

- Offer HIV PrEP and doxy PEP when appropriate.
- Encourage routine STI screening and positive sexual health practices.

DISCLOSURES

The author has nothing to disclose.

REFERENCES

1. Ronald AR, Alfa MJ. Microbiology of the genitourinary system. In: Baron S, editor. Medical microbiology. 4th edition. Galveston (TX): University of Texas Medical Branch at Galveston; 1996. Chapter 97. PMID: 21413302.
2. Holmes KK, Sparling PF, Stamm WE, et al. Sexually transmitted diseases. 4th edition. New York: McGraw Hill Professional; 2007.
3. Singh AE, Romanowski B. Syphilis: review with emphasis on clinical, epidemiologic, and some biologic features. Clin Microbiol Rev 1999;12(2):187–209.
4. Stephanie E, Cohen MD, Jeffrey D, et al. Syphilis in the modern era. Infectious Disease Clinics of North America 2013;27(4):705–22.
5. Centers for Disease Control and Prevention (CDC), Congenital syphilis, Available at: https://www.cdc.gov/std/treatment-guidelines/congenital-syphilis.htm (Accessed 25 August 2024).
6. McDonald R, O'Callaghan K, Torrone E, et al. Vital signs: missed opportunities for preventing congenital syphilis — United States, 2022. MMWR Morb Mortal Wkly Rep 2023;72:1269–74.
7. Centers for Disease Control and Prevention (CDC), National Overview of STIs, Available at: https://www.cdc.gov/sti-statistics/annual/index.html (Accessed 23 November 2024), 2023.
8. Centers for Disease Control and Prevention (CDC), Syphilis surveillance supplemental Slides 2018-2022, Available at: https://www.cdc.gov/sti-statistics/syphilis-supplement/index.html (Accessed 25 August 2024).
9. Ethics ratings of nearly all professions down in U.S, Available at: https://news.gallup.com/poll/608903/ethics-ratings-nearly-professions-down.aspx (Accessed 25 August 2024), 2024.
10. Centers for Disease Control and Prevention (CDC), Guide to taking a sexual history, Available at: https://www.cdc.gov/sti/hcp/clinical-guidance/taking-a-sexual-history.html (Accessed 25 August 2024).
11. Papp JR, Park IU, Fakile Y, et al. CDC laboratory Recommendations for syphilis testing, United States, 2024. MMWR Recomm Rep (Morb Mortal Wkly Rep) 2024;73(1):1–32.
12. Workowski KA, Bachmann LH, Chan PA, et al. Sexually transmitted infections treatment guidelines, 2021. MMWR Recomm Rep (Morb Mortal Wkly Rep) 2021;70(4):1–187.
13. National Academies of Sciences, Engineering, and Medicine. Sexually transmitted infections: adopting a sexual health paradigm. Washington, DC: The National Academies Press; 2021.
14. Lynn WA, Lightman S. Syphilis and HIV: a dangerous combination. Lancet Infect Dis 2004;4(7):456–66.
15. Bachmann LH, Barbee LA, Chan P, et al. CDC clinical guidelines on the use of doxycycline postexposure prophylaxis for bacterial sexually transmitted infection prevention, United States, 2024. MMWR Recomm Rep (Morb Mortal Wkly Rep) 2024;73(RR-2):1–8.

Current Challenges in Gonorrhea Management
A Focus on Diagnosis, Treatment, and Antimicrobial Resistance

Gabriel Lee, BS[a], Matt F. Hoffman, DNP, APRN, FNP-C[b],
Courtney DuBois Shihabuddin, DNP, APRN-CNP, AGPCNP-BC[c],*

KEYWORDS

- Gonorrhea • *Neisseria gonorrhoeae* • Antimicrobial resistance • Sexual health
- Sexually transmitted infections (STIs) • Men who have sex with men (MSM)
- LGBTQIA2+ • Expedited partner therapy (EPT)

KEY POINTS

- Gonorrhea remains the second most common bacterial sexually transmitted infection in the United States, with 1.57 million new cases annually, requiring targeted public health interventions.
- The emergence of drug-resistant *Neisseria gonorrhoeae* poses significant challenges, necessitating updates in treatment protocols, particularly for at-risk populations like men who have sex with men and lesbian, gay, bisexual, transgender, queer, intersex, asexual, and 2 Spirit+ communities.
- Enhanced diagnostic accuracy through extragenital testing and comprehensive sexual health histories is crucial for detecting asymptomatic gonorrhea, especially in high-risk groups.
- Ceftriaxone remains the primary treatment of gonorrhea, but ongoing resistance trends emphasize the need for continued monitoring and updated clinical guidelines.
- Implementing expedited partner therapy is critical to preventing reinfection and reducing transmission, underscoring the importance of patient education and adherence.

[a] College of Medicine, Ohio State University, 1645 Neil Avenue, Columbus, OH 43210, USA; [b] School of Nursing, Round Rock College of Nursing, Texas A&M University, 3950 North AW Grimes Boulevard, Round Rock, TX 78665, USA; [c] Adult-Gerontology Primary Care Nurse Practitioner Program, Adult-Gerontology Clinical Nurse Specialist Program, The Columbus Free Clinic, The Ohio State University-College of Nursing, 395 Newton Hall, 295 West 10th Avenue, Columbus, OH 43210-1289, USA
* Corresponding author. The Ohio State University College of Nursing, 395 Newton Hall, 295 West 10th Avenue, Columbus, OH 43210.
E-mail address: shihabuddin.2@osu.edu

Nurs Clin N Am 60 (2025) 537–552
https://doi.org/10.1016/j.cnur.2024.10.005   nursing.theclinics.com

In the United States, it is estimated that there are 1,568,000 new *Neisseria gonorrhoeae* infections annually, making gonorrhea the second most frequently reported bacterial infectious disease.[1] Gonococcal infections, such as urethritis, cervicitis, epididymitis, and proctitis, contribute significantly to health complications among sexually active individuals. The management of these sexually transmitted infections (STIs) has progressed overtime, primarily in response to the growing issue of antibiotic resistance.

PATHOPHYSIOLOGY OF GONORRHEA AND/CLINICAL MANIFESTATIONS

Gonorrhea is an STI caused by the bacterium *N gonorrhoeae*. The bacterium can adhere to and invade the mucosal surfaces of the genitourinary tract, rectum, pharynx, and conjunctiva. This adherence and invasion are mediated by pili and outer membrane proteins that facilitate attachment to host cells and evasion of the host immune response. Once attached, the gonorrhea bacterium invades the epithelial cells, avoiding initial immune detection. The invasion of epithelial cells triggers an inflammatory response. This response is characterized by the recruitment of neutrophils to the site of infection, resulting in the purulent discharge commonly associated with gonorrhea.[2] The inflammation can cause tissue damage, leading to symptoms such as urethritis in patients assigned male at birth (AMAB) men and cervicitis in patients who are assigned female at birth (AFAB).

In AFAB patients, the cervix is the primary site of infection by *N gonorrhoeae* in people with uteri. A significant proportion of AFAB patients with cervical gonococcal infection, reaching up to 70% in certain studies, remain asymptomatic.[3] Because AFAB patients are primarily asymptomatic, determining the incubation period can be hard to pinpoint. When genital symptoms do occur, they typically present within 10 days post-exposure.[4] Symptomatic infections are often characterized by vaginal pruritus and/or mucopurulent discharge. Some patients may experience spotting between menstrual cycles or menorrhagia. Pain is generally not observed unless there is an upper genital tract infection, where symptoms such as abdominal pain and dyspareunia may prompt patients to seek clinical evaluation.[5] The cervixes may appear normal or have overt discharge from the cervical os upon visual examination. The cervical mucosa is frequently friable. It is important to note that clinical manifestations of gonococcal cervical infection are often indistinguishable from those caused by acute cervicitis of other etiologies.[6] Pelvic inflammatory disease (PID) develops in about 10% to 20% of AFAB patients with cervical gonorrhea; *N gonorrhoeae* is identified as the causative agent in approximately 40% of PID cases.[7]

In AMAB patients, *N gonorrhoeae* results in urethritis and epididymitis. AMAB patients with gonococcal urethritis may exhibit a range of symptoms. The discharge, often spontaneously visible at the urethral meatus, tends to be purulent or mucopurulent and can be copious. Complications of gonococcal urethritis can include penile lymphangitis, penile edema ("bull-headed clap"), periurethral abscesses, and rarely, post-inflammatory urethral strictures.[8] Acute unilateral epididymitis can arise as a complication of gonococcal infection, although it is more frequently caused by *Chlamydia trachomatis*, particularly in patients aged under 35 years.[9] Epididymal infections often involve gonococcal and chlamydial pathogens rather than *N gonorrhoeae* alone.

AMAB patients with epididymitis may present with unilateral testicular pain and swelling. This is often elicited by obtaining a patient history and completing a physical examination. Additional diagnostic tests may be necessary to differentiate infectious epididymitis from other causes of acute testicular pain, such as testicular torsion or trauma.

N gonorrhoeae is a local infection that can infect the rectum and pharynx, but these infections are usually asymptomatic. Occasionally, the bacteria can spread from a mucosal site through the bloodstream, leading to a disseminated infection. Furthermore, *N gonorrhoeae* can cause a severe form of conjunctivitis in adults and adolescents, which can be transmitted through nonsexual contact.[10]

GENERAL IMPORTANCE OF SEXUAL HEALTH HISTORY AND BEST PRACTICES

An adequate sexual health history may function similarly to preventive care measures in that it allows clinicians an opportunity to identify behaviors and high-risk practices with high incidences of morbidity and mortality.[11] Literature continues to examine sexual health history from multiple perspectives, such as approaches to student education, barriers to implementation, effective and patient-centered approaches, as well as settings and patient contexts in which a sexual health history should be taken.[12]

Due to the nature of the content and questions discussed when taking a sexual history, there may be thoughts and feelings of anxiety or fear of judgment stemming from variables such as previous clinical experiences, gender, and social and cultural factors. Acknowledging and normalizing these feelings can be beneficial in developing a trusting patient–clinician rapport.[12]

The value of a sexual health history is optimized when combined with a thorough history of present illness and physical examination. Given the variety of clinical settings and patient complaints during which a sexual history may be applicable, an abbreviated screening, at minimum, and awareness of patient sexual practices can provide valuable information when considering differential diagnoses.[13–15] Utilizing best practices and routinely incorporating sexual health information into preventive and acute care visits, regardless of sexual dysfunction complaints, allows clinicians to identify existing risk factors as well as further educational and counseling needs.[16]

It is common in many clinical settings to gather a patient's medical history at the time of their initial visit. Standardized information gathered commonly includes the patient demographics, active and past medical history, surgical history, medications and allergies, social and sexual history, family history, and preventive care practices.[17] The convenience of template forms may inadvertently inhibit a thorough sexual health history and vary across providers based on multiple factors such as educational training, system/organizational expectations, and blank spaces on an electronic health record template.[13,17,18] Although opportunities for alterations to existing processes and forms may not exist, evaluating environment/clinician-specific barriers and opportunities within the electronic health record (EHR) and practice gaps exist across settings.[15]

Among the existing literature containing tips, techniques, and recommendations for taking a sexual health history, the best practices identified share broad commonalities with slight variation based on the patient presentation and nature of the visit.[13–15,17–20] Regardless, taking a sexual health history requires sensitivity, respect, and a nonjudgmental approach to ensure that patients feel comfortable discussing intimate details.[19,20]

Best practices emphasized throughout the literature include using inclusive, gender-neutral language and normalizing sexual health conversations as part of routine care to reduce stigma.[15,19,21] It is important to ask open-ended questions to gather information about sexual behaviors, partners, contraception use, and STI risk without making assumptions based on appearance or identity.[11,15,18] Establishing trust through confidentiality and explaining the relevance of questions help create a safe environment. Active listening, neutral demeanor, and cultural competence ensure

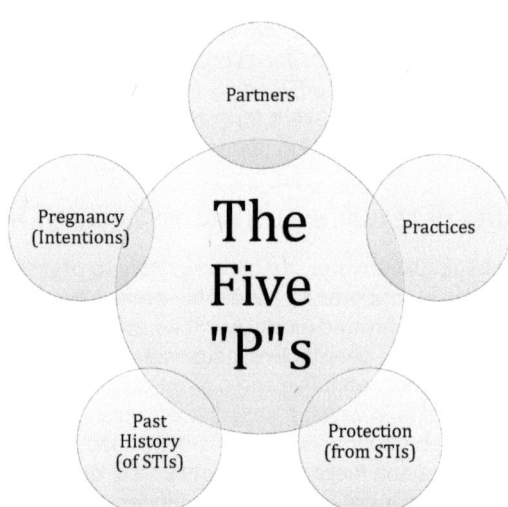

Fig. 1. The 5 P's framework for taking a sexual history. (*Data from* Centers for Disease Control and Prevention. A Guide to Taking a Sexual History.; 2024:24. https://www.cdc.gov/std/treatment/SexualHistory.htm (does not require permission).[1])

all patients feel respected, regardless of their background or experiences.[14,15,19,21] Current education for clinicians focuses on using the "Five P's" and nuanced approaches based on the practice setting and patient-centered needs[19,20] (**Fig. 1**).

AT-RISK POPULATIONS
Young Adults

In 2022, over 31 million young adults, aged 18 to 24 years, lived in the United States.[22] Young adults are at significantly higher risk for STIs, including *N gonorrhoeae*, with about half of reported STIs occurring in this population.[23] A retrospective study in Pennsylvania analyzed gonorrhea and chlamydia among adolescents and young adults from 2004 to 2014 and found that the rate of STI acquisition was significantly higher among female-identifying patients, with patients living at or below 185% of the national poverty line having higher rates of chlamydia and gonorrhea.[24] Multiple risk factors contribute to young adults having higher rates of STIs, including condomless sex, multiple sexual partners, and having sex while intoxicated or high.[25]

Another contributing factor is the presence or lack of sexual education in schooling. A systematic review of systematic reviews of sexual education programs demonstrated that these types of interventions have been proven to be effective at reducing high-risk sexual behaviors. This kind of education is also essential, with abstinence-focused education being less effective at improving sexual behaviors.[26] Additionally, sex education programs are not standardized in the United States, with one study citing inconsistencies between programs across the country.[27] These factors contribute to young adults having higher rates of STI acquisition and, more specifically, increasing gonorrhea infection rates among young adults, making this population a necessary population to target for educational and harm reduction interventions.

TESTING CONSIDERATIONS

Young adults should be offered asymptomatic and symptomatic STI testing as STIs can present with or without symptoms in both male and female-identifying patients.[28]

Additionally, pharyngeal gonorrhea testing has been demonstrated to be necessary, especially among young adults.[29] A case–control study from 2012 to 2014 examined 245 young adults attending one of 12 STI clinics in Los Angeles who reported giving oral sex to a partner within the past 90 days. The study demonstrated that 28% of gonorrhea cases would have been missed without pharyngeal testing.[29] With the increased risk factors for STI transmission among young adults, it is imperative that comprehensive asymptomatic and symptomatic STI testing be offered to all patients.

Older Adults

Older adults are another population that has been experiencing a rise in gonorrhea infections in the past decade. STIs have increased substantially in recent years among older adults, with gonorrhea rates more than doubling from 2007 to 2017.[30] With increases in life expectancy, older adults continue to be sexually active later in life, with one review emphasizing that many AFAB patients and AMAB patients remain sexually active into their 70s and 80s.[31] While some risk factors are similar in older adults compared to the general population, one study compared the risk factors of older adults compared to younger adults in Baltimore, Maryland, from 2011 to 2016.[32] Older adults were more likely to report "never" using condoms, binge drinking (4–5 drinks in one sitting in the last 30 days), sex with alcohol, cocaine use, intravenous drug use, and exchanging sex for money, drugs, or other goods compared to younger adults.[31] Older AFAB patients were also more likely to report being a victim of sexual assault compared to younger AFAB patients.[32]

Swingers

An additional consideration among older adults is the rising popularity of swingers. Swingers are typically members of a heterosexual couple who have sex with other couples and/or singles in the swingers subculture.[33] While not much data are available to depict the number of adults who are a part of the swingers subculture, swingers are a hidden but vital population to consider in STI prevention. A significant issue is self-identification in clinical spaces. From 2009 to 2012, one STI clinic in the Netherlands surveyed 289 adults whose behaviors aligned with the definition of swinging. Overall, 44% of patients did not identify as a swinger despite their behaviors aligning with the definition. Additionally, this clinic saw a 13% STI positivity rate, with 57% of respondents reporting condomless sex during vaginal sex.[33]

An additional study found that swingers were more likely to underestimate the STI status of their partners, further contributing to STI transmission among this population.[34] Additionally, swingers comprised a higher percentage of STI-positive results than men who have sex with men (MSM) in one Dutch clinic.[35] At this clinic, older swingers had a 4% gonorrhea positivity rate. Overall, swingers represent an essential yet hidden population that requires crucial clinical consideration in STI management.

Lesbian, Gay, Bisexual, Transgender, Queer, Intersex, Asexual, and 2 Spirit+

Lesbian, gay, bisexual, transgender, queer, intersex, asexual, and 2 Spirit (LGBTQIA2+) individuals are disproportionately affected by STIs, including gonorrhea. One study analyzed the rates of gonorrhea and chlamydia MSM and men who do not have sex with men in San Francisco and found that from 1999 to 2008, 72% of gonorrhea infections were in MSM.[36] Another study analyzing patients who participated in extragenital sexual activity from January 2012 to October 2014 also concluded that MSM had the highest rates of gonorrhea compared to other groups.[37] Risk factors can contribute to these rates and often appear earlier in LGBTQIA2+ identifying patients. One study indicates that STI risk factors such as the number of sexual partners, concurrent sexual partners, and age of first sexual experience were higher among bisexual-identified adolescents compared to heterosexual youth MSM and gay-identifying respondents, and these behaviors can present earlier in life and can vary among sexual orientation and sexual behaviors.[38]

Additionally, AFAB patients who have sex with both men and women WSB men and women were significantly more likely to report more sexual partners, were more likely to engage in transactional sex, and were more likely to report drug and alcohol use, contributing to their equal or higher rates of test positivity for all STIs except urogenital chlamydia compared to AFAB patients who have sex with men (WSM). AFAB patients who have sex with AFAB patients women who have sex with women (WSW) had a lower rate of gonorrhea test positivity compared to WSB and WSM.[39]

Sex Workers

Sex workers are at higher risk for contracting gonorrhea due to multiple behavioral and structural reasons. Sex workers are defined as any individual who exchanges sexual acts for a form of compensation, including but not limited to money, drugs, and other services.[40] A Maryland-based study demonstrated that involvement in sex work among cisgender female sex workers predicted the incidence of gonorrhea infections. Sexual violence was also a predictor of gonorrhea infections among cisgender female sex workers.[41] Unfortunately, sex workers experience disproportionate rates of sexual violence, which is further exacerbated by the lack of legal protections for sex workers, causing sexual violence cases to go unmonitored and unreported.[42] Additionally, sex workers are more likely to have inconsistent condom use (ICU), which is the proximal risk of transmission and infection, with one study reporting 39.2% of sex workers having recent ICU. Many factors contribute to ICU among sex workers, including client coercion, the number of clients, and client intoxication.[43]

MISCONCEPTIONS ABOUT PREVENTATIVE HEALTH CARE AND RISK
Pre-exposure Prophylaxis

Among specific patient populations, perceptions of medication use like pre-exposure prophylaxis (PrEP) and birth control have been correlated with a decrease in the use of barrier protection, such as condoms. One descriptive retrospective study in Madrid, Spain, conducted interviews with 110 PrEP users over 2 years, from 2017 to 2019, to ascertain factors associated with PrEP usage and adherence, including condom usage. The study found a statistically significant decrease in condom usage before and after initiating PrEP. While there were no substantial changes in gonorrhea rates before and after initiating PrEP,[44] the lack of condom usage increases the risk for STI acquisition, suggesting a need for reinforced patient education during PrEP visits. Another study analyzed condom use and PrEP uptake in MSM from 2014 to 2017 in San Francisco and estimated that while PrEP usage increased from 9.8% to 44.7%, condom usage decreased from 18.5% to 9.4%.[45]

Birth Control

One study in Northern California surveyed 1194 AFAB patients aged 15 to 24 years attending a family planning clinic and distributed 3, 6, and 12-month surveys after initiating a form of hormonal contraception.[46] The study found that condom use decreased by 27%, suggesting a need for reinforced patient education. The Centers for Disease Control and Prevention (CDC) utilized the Youth Risk Behavior Study and found that only 9% of high school students had used condoms if they had some form of contraception such as an intrauterine device or birth control pills.[47] Considering that an individual AFAB's likelihood of becoming pregnant is one-half the possibility of contracting gonorrhea from an infected partner, these data suggest that more education is necessary to discuss the impact of birth control and condom use on gonorrhea and STI prevention.[48]

Current Neisseria gonorrhoeae Treatment Guidelines

Annual screening for *N gonorrhoeae* is recommended for all sexually active AFAB patients aged under 25 years and for older AFAB patients who are at increased risk of infection. This includes AFAB patients aged 25 years and older with a new sex partner, multiple sex partners, a partner with concurrent partners, or a partner with an STI. Additional risk factors for gonorrhea include ICU among nonmonogamous individuals, a history of STIs, and exchanging sex for money or drugs.

Clinicians should consider the specific communities they serve and consult local public health authorities for guidance on identifying high-risk groups, as gonococcal infections are often concentrated in specific geographic locations and neighborhoods. MSM are at high risk for gonococcal infection, or those at risk for human immunodeficiency virus (HIV) should be screened at the appropriate anatomic sites of exposure (per a review of the patient's sexual history) every 3 to 6 months, with at least annual screening recommended for all MSM. Screening for gonorrhea in heterosexual men and AFAB patients over 25 years who are at low risk for infection is not recommended. Additionally, recent travel history with sexual contacts outside the United States should be included in gonorrhea evaluations[1] (**Box 1**).

Box 1
Treatment guidelines for gonococcal infection

Recommended Regimen for Uncomplicated Gonococcal Infection of the Cervix, Urethra, or Rectum Among Adults and Adolescents[1]
    Ceftriaxone 500 mg[a] IM in a single dose for persons weighing less than 150 kg
    If chlamydial infection has not been excluded, treat for chlamydia with doxycycline 100 mg orally 2 times/day for 7 days.

Alternative regimens
    If cephalosporin allergy:
        Gentamicin 240 mg IM in a single dose
        PLUS
        Azithromycin 2 g orally in a single dose
    If ceftriaxone administration is not available or not feasible:
        Cefixime 800 mg[b] orally in a single dose

Recommended regimen for uncomplicated gonococcal infection of the pharynx among adolescents and adults
    Ceftriaxone 500 mg[c] IM in a single dose for persons weighing less than 150 kg

[a]For persons weighing 150 kg or more, 1 g ceftriaxone should be administered. [b]If chlamydial infection has not been excluded, providers should treat for chlamydia with doxycycline 100 mg orally 2 times/day for 7 days. [c]For persons weighing 150 kg or more, 1 g ceftriaxone should be administered.

Data from Centers for Disease Control and Prevention. Gonococcal infections among adolescents and adults - STI treatment guidelines. Sexually Transmitted Infections Treatment Guidelines, 2021. December 5, 2022. Accessed September 17, 2024. https://www.cdc.gov/std/treatment-guidelines/gonorrhea-adults.htm (does not require permission).

GONORRHEA RESISTANCE AND THE IMPORTANCE OF SCREENING/TREATMENT

N gonorrhoeae is increasingly resistant to many common antimicrobial drugs,[49] presenting a significant global health threat. This rise in antimicrobial resistance (AMR) could lead to a hidden epidemic, exacerbating the current situation. Historically, gonorrheal infections were easily treatable, but they have progressively developed resistance to medications such as penicillin, ciprofloxacin, and azithromycin. Consequently, ceftriaxone remains the sole reliable option for initial treatment. Immediate and effective management strategies are essential to prevent serious outcomes, including infertility and PID, which can result from delayed treatment.

Treatment Failure

Cephalosporin treatment failure occurs when N gonorrhoeae infection persists despite receiving the recommended cephalosporin therapy, indicating a possible cephalosporin-resistant strain. This is especially true in individuals whose partners were also treated and who have a low risk of reinfection. Such failures have been observed in those treated with oral and injectable cephalosporins.

Treatment failure should be suspected in individuals whose symptoms do not resolve within 3 to 5 days after treatment and who report no sexual contact during the posttreatment follow-up period. It should also be suspected in those with a positive test of cure (positive culture after more than 72 hours or positive nucleic acid amplification test [NAAT] after more than 7 days following treatment) when no sexual contact is reported during the follow-up. Additionally, treatment failure should be considered for individuals with a positive culture on the test of cure, particularly if antimicrobial susceptibility testing shows decreased susceptibility to cephalosporins, regardless of reported sexual contact during the follow-up period.

For individuals suspected of experiencing cephalosporin treatment failure, the treating provider should seek guidance from an infectious disease specialist, the National Network of sexually transmitted disease (STD) Clinical Prevention Training Center clinical consultation line, the local or state health department STI program, or the CDC. This consultation is necessary for advice on obtaining cultures, antimicrobial susceptibility testing, and treatment. Suspected treatment failures must be reported to the CDC through the local or state health department within 24 hours of diagnosis.

Patients with suspected treatment failures (**Box 2**) should be retreated with the initial regimen (ceftriaxone 500 mg IM), adding doxycycline if chlamydia infection is present,

---

Box 2
Treatment of suspected cephalosporin treatment failure

Recommended treatment with suspected treatment failures[1]

Retreat with the initial regimen used (ceftriaxone 500 mg IM), with the addition of doxycycline if chlamydia infection exists

Clinical specimens should be obtained for culture (preferably with simultaneous NAAT) and antimicrobial susceptibility testing before retreatment.

Dual treatment with single doses of IM gentamicin 240 mg plus oral azithromycin 2 g when isolates are identified as having elevated cephalosporin MICs

Data from Centers for Disease Control and Prevention. Gonococcal infections among adolescents and adults - STI treatment guidelines. Sexually Transmitted Infections Treatment Guidelines, 2021. December 5, 2022. Accessed September 17, 2024. https://www.cdc.gov/std/treatment-guidelines/gonorrhea-adults.htm (does not require permission).

as reinfections are more common than actual treatment failures. If there is a higher likelihood of treatment failure than reinfection, relevant clinical specimens should be collected for culture (preferably with simultaneous NAAT) and antimicrobial susceptibility testing before retreatment. Dual treatment with a single dose of intramuscular (IM) gentamicin 240 mg plus oral azithromycin 2 g may be considered if isolates have elevated cephalosporin minimum inhibitory concentration (MICs).

For those who experience treatment failure after an alternative regimen (cefixime or gentamicin), ceftriaxone 500 mg as a single IM dose should be administered, with or without an antichlamydial agent, based on chlamydia infection status. A test of cure should be performed 7 to 14 days after retreatment at relevant clinical sites, using culture as the recommended test, preferably with simultaneous NAAT and antimicrobial susceptibility testing *if N gonorrhoeae* is isolated. Clinicians must ensure that the patient's sexual partners from the past 60 days are promptly evaluated with culture and presumptively treated using the same regimen administered to the patients.

Follow-up

Repeat testing for those diagnosed with uncomplicated urogenital or rectal gonorrhea is not necessary if treated with the recommended or alternative regimens. However, individuals with pharyngeal gonorrhea should return for a test of cure within 7 to 14 days posttreatment using culture or NAAT, with the caution that testing at 7 days may increase the likelihood of false positives. If NAAT results are positive, a confirmatory culture should be attempted before retreatment, especially if no culture was previously taken. All positive cultures from the test of cure should undergo antimicrobial susceptibility testing. Persistent symptoms after treatment should be evaluated using culture (with or without simultaneous NAAT) and antimicrobial susceptibility testing. Additionally, other organisms may be responsible for persistent urethritis, cervicitis, or proctitis.[1]

DOXY AS POST-EXPOSURE PROPHYLAXIS

The use of doxycycline as post-exposure prophylaxis (doxy PEP) represents an innovative, patient-controlled strategy for preventing STIs in specific populations. In June 2024, the CDC issued a statement advising MSM and transgender AFAB patients, through shared decision-making with health care providers, to be given a prescription for doxy PEP, to be taken within 72 hours after engaging in oral, vaginal, or anal sex to prevent infection of bacterial STIs (gonorrhea, chlamydia, syphilis). The advised dosage is 200 mg, with a maximum limit of 200 mg every 24 hours.[50] Anyone diagnosed with gonorrhea should also be screened for other STIs, such as chlamydia, syphilis, and HIV. Individuals who test negative for HIV should be offered HIV PrEP.

CASE STUDY OF PHARYNGEAL GONORRHEA INFECTIOUS WITHOUT SEXUAL CONTACT IN THE UNIVERSITY SETTING

A 19 year old Caucasian cisgender female (she/her) presented with no known drug allergies (**Table 1**). Her current medication includes fexofenadine 180 mg, taken once daily for seasonal allergies. Her past medical history is notable for seasonal allergies, and she has no history of surgical procedures. She is a full-time college student and reports consuming an occasional glass of wine monthly. She denies both current and previous use of tobacco or recreational drugs. She resides in on-campus housing and identifies as heterosexual. She recently started dating a cisgender male and reports being a virgin with no history of STIs. Her family history is unremarkable.

Table 1
Pertinent medical history, assessment findings, and diagnostics

Patient Information	
Age and Sex	19 year old cisgender female
Allergies	No Known Drug Allergies
Medication	Fexofenadine 60 mg, 1 tablet daily
Past Medical History	• Seasonal allergies • No surgical history • No previous hospitalizations
Social History	• Full-time college student; lives in on-campus dorms • Reports 1–2 glasses of wine monthly • Negative for vaping, tobacco, and recreational drug use • Denies ever having intercourse or history of STIs • In a new monogamous relationship with cisgender male
Family History	• Both parents alive and well; no remarkable medical history • Older sister alive and well; no remarkable medical history
Assessment Findings and Diagnostics	
Pertinent Positives	• Swollen cervical lymph nodes • Erythematous pharynx
Pertinent Negatives	• No cough or nasal congestion • Absence of genitourinary complaints
Diagnostic Testing	• Positive: throat/pharynx culture (*N gonorrhea*) • Negative: urine NG/C • Negative: Serum hCG

These data are specific to the case study in the study; therefore, no reference is necessary.

Case History

The patient presents to the university student health center with complaints of a 3 week history of a sore, itchy throat, occasional pain with swallowing, and swollen lymph nodes following a complete course of azithromycin prescribed by primary care provider (PCP).

The patient reports initially attributing symptoms to seasonal weather changes since she commonly experiences nasal congestion and sore throat at the beginning of each fall season. Although she was not experiencing symptoms of congestion, she began fexofenadine 60 mg daily. Within 1 week, she did not experience any change in symptoms. After searching her symptoms online, she considered the possibility of mononucleosis or strep since she recently started a new relationship approximately 1 week before the onset of symptoms.

After 1 week of continued symptoms, she was seen by her PCP for evaluation and treatment of continued symptoms. At that time, her throat was swabbed at the clinic and was negative for streptococcus A via a rapid Strep A test. Along with recommendations for supportive care with over-the-counter analgesics, a one time course of azithromycin was sent to her pharmacy with instructions to fill and complete within 24 to 48 hours if symptoms did not improve or resolve. Upon completing the course of antibiotics, the symptoms persisted and remained unchanged, resulting in her visit to the university student health clinic.

Upon review of the patient's chart, the student health clinician asked the patient what kinds of sex she was having, to which the patient denied penetrative vaginal or anal intercourse but endorsed performing and receiving oral sex with her new boyfriend. With this new information, the clinician proceeded with a more detailed risk assessment of the patient and the new partner's sexual histories and risk factors.

After determining the patient's risk and lack of detailed information regarding her partner's sexual history, the patient was counseled regarding the possible differential diagnoses, including risk for pharyngeal gonococcal infection. The patient consented to diagnostic testing, including screening for chlamydia and gonorrhea using a NAAT via a pharyngeal swab.

Treatment Plan

The patient should receive a one time dose of ceftriaxone 500 mg administered intramuscularly in the clinic and doxycycline 100 mg taken orally twice daily for 7 days. Expedited partner therapy (EPT)[1,51] should be initiated as legally permitted by applicable statutes and regulations. Key patient education points should emphasize the importance of completing the entire course of antibiotics, disposing of toothbrushes and any other reusable dental hygiene products, and avoiding all sexual activity, including kissing, until antibiotic therapy is completed and a negative test of cure is confirmed. Additionally, patients should be informed of the relevant reporting requirements to the state health department as legally permitted by existing statutes/regulations.[51,52]

Expected Outcome of the Treatment Plan

Following the treatment plan for uncomplicated gonococcal infection of the pharynx as described earlier, the patient is expected to achieve complete resolution of infection and associated secondary symptoms. The most significant potential causes of treatment plan failure involve the patient and/or partner's compliance with completing the full course of antibiotics and strict adherence to avoiding sexual activity/behaviors that put them at risk for reinfection.

DISCUSSION

In all clinical settings, comprehensive differential diagnoses and thorough patient–provider communication are critical components to mitigate variables that may prevent and/or delay appropriate diagnostic testing, diagnosis, and treatment. Contributing factors within the case are identified and discussed later with recommendations.

Past Medical and Social History

Given the patient's medical history, it is reasonable for a recurrence of seasonal allergy symptoms to be considered and addressed with the initial symptom presentation. Additionally, it is prudent for clinicians to consider any new additions to medical and social history, such as new relationships and/or sexual partners. This information should serve as a trigger for initiating sexual history screening, not only as a part of routine care but also as part of new symptoms or findings also seen in STIs.[13,20]

Patient–Provider Rapport

An established rapport benefits the patient and provider. However, a positive relationship does not guarantee transparency and full disclosure on behalf of the patient. When patients seek care across multiple settings, meeting and interacting with a new provider may inhibit or enhance their comfort and/or willingness to share pertinent findings. This is particularly relevant in situations among marginalized groups, such as LGBTQIA2+ patients without access to safe clinical spaces.[15,53] However, hesitation to disclose relevant information may also be seen when a patient feels reluctant or does not wish to disclose information such as a suspected STI to an established provider.

Clarification of Sexual Practices

The use of established practices and algorithms for screening and asking individuals questions about sexual history and sexual practices allows for clear communication, normalizing the conversation along with assurance of confidentiality. As seen from the case earlier, although the patient self-reported being a virgin, she later endorses participating in oral sex with her new partner. Asking specific questions about sexual practices provides clinicians with a better understanding of the individual's sexual behaviors, risks, topics for further teaching, as well as potential preventive care interventions.[13,18]

SUMMARY

Obtaining a thorough sexual health history is critical in delivering comprehensive care and accurately diagnosing STIs such as gonorrhea. Sexual health assessments should be inclusive, asking patients about a variety of sexual behaviors, orientations, and practices without assumption or judgment. This helps to identify individuals at risk who may otherwise not be screened or treated appropriately, as many STIs can be asymptomatic or present with nonspecific symptoms.

Regular and appropriate screening is essential, particularly for high-risk populations, to ensure early detection and reduce the risk of complications or transmission. Clinicians must stay informed about evolving screening guidelines to capture infections that traditional approaches might miss. Moreover, AMR in *N gonorrhoeae* continues to challenge treatment efforts. Updated treatment regimens and partner management strategies are essential to prevent reinfection and control the spread of resistant strains. Ongoing surveillance and adherence to treatment guidelines, combined with targeted health education efforts, are critical in combating the rise of gonorrhea and ensuring effective management of STIs.

CLINICS CARE POINTS

- Comprehensive sexual histories
  Always obtain a thorough sexual health history, including questions about oral and anal sex, to ensure appropriate extragenital testing and accurate diagnosis of gonorrhea.
- Extragenital screening
  Encourage extragenital testing (pharyngeal and rectal swabs) in high-risk populations, particularly MSM, as many gonorrhea infections in these sites can be asymptomatic.
- Overreliance on symptoms
  Relying solely on symptoms may lead to missed diagnoses, as up to 70% of gonorrhea infections, especially in women and MSM, can be asymptomatic.
- EPT
  Offer EPT to patients with gonorrhea, which allows treatment of sexual partners without a clinical visit, reducing reinfection and ongoing transmission (state laws vary).
- Delayed treatment adjustments
  Delaying treatment updates due to evolving AMR trends may lead to therapeutic failure. Stay updated on local resistance patterns and national guidelines.

DECLARATION OF AI AND AI-ASSISTED TECHNOLOGIES IN THE WRITING PROCESS

During the preparation of this work the author(s) used generative artificial intelligence (AI) in order to write the article. After using this tool/service, the author(s) reviewed and edited the content as needed and take(s) full responsibility for the content of the publication.

DISCLOSURE

The authors have nothing to disclose.

REFERENCES

1. Centers for Disease Control and Prevention. Gonococcal infections among adolescents and adults - STI treatment guidelines. Sexually Transmitted Infections Treatment Guidelines 2021. Available at: https://www.cdc.gov/std/treatment-guidelines/gonorrhea-adults.htm. Accessed September 17, 2024.
2. Edwards JL, Butler EK. The pathobiology of Neisseria gonorrhoeae lower female genital tract infection. Front Microbiol 2011;2:102.
3. McCormack WM, Stumacher RJ, Johnson K, et al. Clinical spectrum of gonococcal infection in women. Lancet Lond Engl 1977;1(8023):1182–5.
4. Platt R, Rice PA, McCormack WM. Risk of acquiring gonorrhea and prevalence of abnormal adnexal findings among women recently exposed to gonorrhea. JAMA 1983;250(23):3205–9.
5. Barlow D, Phillips I. Gonorrhoea in women. Diagnostic, clinical, and laboratory aspects. Lancet Lond Engl 1978;1(8067):761–4.
6. Iqbal U, Wills C. Cervicitis. In: StatPearls. StatPearls Publishing; 2024. Available at: http://www.ncbi.nlm.nih.gov/books/NBK562193/. Accessed September 22, 2024.
7. Eschenbach DA, Buchanan TM, Pollock HM, et al. Polymicrobial etiology of acute pelvic inflammatory disease. N Engl J Med 1975;293(4):166–71.
8. Sherrard J, Barlow D. Gonorrhoea in men: clinical and diagnostic aspects. Genitourin Med 1996;72(6):422–6.
9. Holmes KK, Berger RE, Alexander ER. Acute epididymitis: etiology and therapy. Arch Androl 1979;3(4):309–16.
10. Zumla A. Mandell, Douglas, and Bennett's principles and practice of infectious diseases. Lancet Infect Dis 2010;10(5):303–4.
11. Bickley L, Szilagyi P, Hoffman R, et al. Bates' Guide to physical examination and history taking. 13th edition. Philadelphia, PA: Lippincott Williams & Wilkins; 2023.
12. Lamb J, Holland L, Mahony A. The importance of taking a sexual health history. Aust Nurs Midwifery J 2018;25(9). Available at: https://www.proquest.com/docview/2390573207?sourcetype=Scholarly%20Journals. Accessed September 17, 2024.
13. Taylor MM, Frasure-Williams J, Burnett P, et al. Interventions to improve sexually transmitted disease screening in clinic-based settings. Sex Transm Dis 2016;43(2 Suppl 1):S28–41.
14. Althof SE, Rosen RC, Perelman MA, et al. Standard operating procedures for taking a sexual history. J Sex Med 2013;10(1):26–35.
15. National LGBT Health Education Center. Taking routine histories of sexual health: a system-wide approach for health centers. The Fenway Institute; 2015. p. 38. Available at: https://www.lgbtqiahealtheducation.org/publication/taking-routine-histories-of-sexual-health-a-system-wide-approach-for-health-centers/download/.
16. Ribeiro S, Alarcão V, Simões R, et al. General practitioners' procedures for sexual history taking and treating sexual dysfunction in primary care. J Sex Med 2014;11(2):386–93.

17. LeBlond RF, Brown DD, Suneja M, et al. History taking and the medical record. In: DeGowin's diagnostic examination. 10th edition. McGraw-Hill Education; 2015. Available at: . Accessed September 17, 2024.
18. Sexual health and your patients: a provider's Guide | NCSH. National coalition for sexual health. Available at: https://nationalcoalitionforsexualhealth.org/tools/for-healthcare-providers/sexual-health-and-your-patients-a-providers-guide. Accessed September 17, 2024.
19. Centers for Disease Control and Prevention. A Guide to taking a sexual history. 2024. Available at: https://www.cdc.gov/std/treatment/SexualHistory.htm.
20. Savoy M, O'Gurek D, Brown-James A. Sexual health history: techniques and tips. Am Fam Physician 2020;101(5):286–93.
21. French K. How to improve your sexual health history-taking skills. Pract Nurse 2010;40(2):27–30.
22. The Annie E. Casey Foundation. Young adult population ages 18 to 24 by race and ethnicity | KIDS COUNT Data Center. Available at: https://datacenter.aecf.org/data/tables/11207-young-adult-population-ages-18-to-24-by-race-and-ethnicity. Accessed September 17, 2024.
23. National overview of STIs. 2022. Available at: https://www.cdc.gov/std/statistics/2022/overview.htm. Accessed September 17, 2024.
24. Pinto CN, Dorn LD, Chinchilli VM, et al. Chlamydia and gonorrhea acquisition among adolescents and young adults in Pennsylvania: a rural and urban comparison. Sex Transm Dis 2018;45(2):99.
25. Rusley JC, Tao J, Koinis-Mitchell D, et al. Trends in risk behaviors and sexually transmitted infections among youth presenting to a sexually transmitted infection clinic in the United States, 2013–2017. Int J STD AIDS 2022;33(7):634.
26. Denford S, Abraham C, Campbell R, et al. A comprehensive review of reviews of school-based interventions to improve sexual-health. Health Psychol Rev 2017; 11(1):33–52.
27. Schmidt SC, Wandersman A, Hills KJ. Evidence-based sexuality education programs in schools: do they align with the national sexuality education standards? Am J Sex Educ 2015;10(2):177–95.
28. Maraynes ME, Chao JH, Agoritsas K, et al. Screening for asymptomatic chlamydia and gonorrhea in adolescent males in an urban pediatric emergency department. World J Clin Pediatr 2017;6(3):154.
29. Javanbakht M, Westmoreland D, Gorbach P. Factors associated with pharyngeal gonorrhea in young people: implications for prevention. Sex Transm Dis 2018; 45(9):588.
30. Smith ML, Bergeron CD, Goltz HH, et al. Sexually transmitted infection knowledge among older adults: psychometrics and test–retest reliability. Int J Environ Res Public Health 2020;17(7):2462.
31. DeLamater J. Sexual expression in later life: a review and synthesis - PubMed. J Sex Res 2012;49(2–3):125–41.
32. Tao X, Ghanem K, Page K, et al. Risk factors predictive of sexually transmitted infection diagnosis in young compared to older patients attending sexually transmitted diseases clinics - pmc. Int J STD AIDS 2020;32(2):142–9.
33. Spauwen LWL, Niekamp AM, Hoebe CJPA, et al. Do swingers self-identify as swingers when attending STI services for testing? A cross-sectional study. Sex Transm Infect 2018;94(8):559–61.
34. Niekamp AM, Spauwen LWL, Dukers-Muijrers NHTM, et al. How aware are swingers about their swing sex partners' risk behaviours, and sexually transmitted infection status? BMC Infect Dis 2021;21(1):172.

35. Dukers-Muijrers NH, Niekamp AM, Brouwers EE, et al. Older and swinging; need to identify hidden and emerging risk groups at STI clinics - PubMed. Sex Transm Infect 2010;86(4):315–7.

36. Scott HM, Bernstein KT, Raymond HF, et al. Racial/ethnic and sexual behavior disparities in rates of sexually transmitted infections, San Francisco, 1999-2008. BMC Publ Health 2010;10:315.

37. Bamberger DM, Graham G, Dennis L, et al. Extragenital gonorrhea and Chlamydia among men and women according to type of sexual exposure. Sex Transm Dis 2019;46(5):329.

38. Everett BG, Schnarrs PW, Rosario M, et al. Sexual orientation disparities in sexually transmitted infection risk behaviors and risk determinants among sexually active adolescent males: results from a school-based sample. Am J Publ Health 2014;104(6):1107–12.

39. Rahman N, Ghanem KG, Gilliams E, et al. Factors associated with sexually transmitted infection diagnosis in women who have sex with women, women who have sex with men and women who have sex with both. Sex Transm Infect 2021;97(6):423–8.

40. Sawicki DA, Meffert BN, Read K, et al. Culturally competent health care for sex workers: an examination of myths that stigmatize sex-work and hinder access to care. Sex Relatsh Ther J Br Assoc Sex Relatsh Ther 2019;34(3):355–71.

41. Park JN, Gaydos CA, White RH, et al. Incidence and predictors of Chlamydia, gonorrhea and trichomonas among a prospective cohort of cisgender female sex workers in Baltimore, Maryland. Sex Transm Dis 2019;46(12):788.

42. Deering KN, Amin A, Shoveller J, et al. A systematic review of the correlates of violence against sex workers. Am J Publ Health 2014;104(5):e42–54.

43. Decker MR, Park JN, Allen ST, et al. Inconsistent condom use among female sex workers: partner-specific influences of substance use, violence, and condom coercion. AIDS Behav 2020;24(3):762–74.

44. Aguirrebengoa OA, García MV, Ramírez DA, et al. Low use of condom and high STI incidence among men who have sex with men in PrEP programs. PLoS One 2021;16(2):e0245925.

45. Chen YH, Guigayoma J, McFarland W, et al. Increases in pre-exposure prophylaxis use and decreases in condom use: behavioral patterns among HIV-negative San Francisco men who have sex with men, 2004–2017. AIDS Behav 2019;23(7):1841–5.

46. Goldstein RL, Upadhyay UD, Raine TR. With pills, patches, rings, and shots: who still uses condoms? A longitudinal cohort study. J Adolesc Health 2013;52(1):77–82.

47. Szucs LE. Condom and contraceptive use among sexually active high school students — youth risk behavior survey, United States, 2019. MMWR Suppl 2020;69. https://doi.org/10.15585/mmwr.su6901a2.

48. Cates WJ, Steiner MJ. Dual protection against unintended pregnancy and sexually transmitted infections: what is the best contraceptive approach? Sex Transm Dis 2002;29(3):168.

49. Omeershffudin UNM, Kumar S. Emerging threat of antimicrobial resistance in Neisseria gonorrhoeae: pathogenesis, treatment challenges, and potential for vaccine development. Arch Microbiol 2023;205(10):330.

50. Bachmann LH. CDC clinical guidelines on the use of doxycycline postexposure prophylaxis for bacterial sexually transmitted infection prevention, United States, 2024. MMWR Recomm Rep (Morb Mortal Wkly Rep) 2024;73. https://doi.org/10.15585/mmwr.rr7302a1.

51. CDC. Duty to warn for health care settings. Sex Transm Infect 2024. Available at: https://www.cdc.gov/sti/hcp/clinical-guidance/duty-to-warn-for-health-care-settings. html. Accessed September 18, 2024.

52. CDC. Legal status of expedited partner therapy (EPT). Sex Transm Infect 2024. Available at: https://www.cdc.gov/sti/php/ept-legal-status/index.html. Accessed September 18, 2024.

53. Lee GA, Fritter J, Shihabuddin CD. Increasing safe clinical spaces and the efforts of clinical research for uninsured and underinsured LGBTQIA2+ patients: a case study of the Rainbow Clinic – a student-run free LGBTQIA2+ clinic. J Clin Transl Sci 2023;7(1):e218.

Diagnosis and Management of Bacterial Prostatitis

Ryan Holley-Mallo, PhD, DNP, NP-C[a,b],*, Jason Gleason, DNP, FNP-C[c,d],
Christopher Gleason, MSN, FNP-C[c,e]

KEYWORDS:

- Urology • Men's health • Prostatitis • Lower urinary tract symptoms (LUTS)

KEY POINTS

- Prostatitis is one of the most common diagnoses faced by men in the United States.
- *Escherichia coli* is the most causative organism responsible for prostatitis infections, but sexually transmitted infections (STIs) and fungal organisms are also responsible for prostatitis infections.
- Nurse practitioners should have a high degree of suspicion for STIs and prescribe antimicrobials with coverage against *Neisseria gonorrhoeae* and *Chlamydia trachomatis* in men who are 35 y of age and younger.
- Alpha blockers, such as terazosin, play a role in the management of prostatitis.
- New and investigative treatments including: botulinum toxin injection, prostatic artery embolization, and transurethral microwave thermotherapy are being studied for their role in the treatment of chronic prostatitis.

INTRODUCTION

Prostatitis is a common complaint faced by men over the age of 18 in the ambulatory setting and is responsible for 5% of all ambulatory visits and 8% of urology visits incurred by men annually.[1] The morbidity sustained by men with regards to prostatitis is nuanced by the fact that there are many forms of prostatitis (**Table 1**) and an intracity of syndromes that each requires specific treatment as outlined by the National Institutes of Health.[2] For the purposes of this article, we will discuss the diagnosis and management of acute and chronic bacterial prostatitis (CBP) within the ambulatory setting. Bacterial prostatitis was once hailed a disease of the urinary tract in older men, but within the United States, it is the most common urinary diagnosis in men

[a] Department of Family & Emergency Medicine Sheridan Community Hospital, 301 North Main Street, Sheridan, MI 48884, USA; [b] Beal University, Bangor, Maine, USA; [c] Primary Care, Veterans Health Administration, Montana, VA, USA; [d] Fitzgerald Health Education Associates By Colilbri; [e] United States Army Reserve
* Corresponding author. Department of Family & Emergency Medicine Sheridan Community Hospital, 301 North Main Street, Sheridan, MI 48884.
E-mail address: RyanMalloDNP@gmail.com

Nurs Clin N Am 60 (2025) 553–561
https://doi.org/10.1016/j.cnur.2024.10.007   nursing.theclinics.com

Table 1
Types of prostatitis

Type	Name	Defined
I	Acute Bacterial Prostatitis	Acute urogenital symptoms with evidence of bacterial infection of the prostate.
II	Chronic Bacterial Prostatitis	Chronic or recurrent urogenital symptoms with evidence of bacterial infection of the prostate.
IIIa	Chronic Prostatitis/ Chronic Pelvic Pain Syndrome - Inflammatory	Chronic or recurrent urogenital symptoms with evidence of inflammation, but not bacterial infection of the prostate.
IIIb	Chronic Prostatitis/Chronic Pelvic Pain Syndrome – Non-Inflammatory	Chronic or recurrent urogenital symptoms without evidence of inflammation or bacterial infection of the prostate; formerly prostatodynia.
IV	Asymptomatic Inflammatory Prostatitis	Absence of urogenital symptoms with evidence of inflammation of the prostate found incidentally.

between the ages of 18 to 50 y[3] and the third most common urinary diagnosis in men over the age of 50 y.[4] Prostatitis is a highly prevalent diagnosis faced by men and one larger United States based research study found the overall prevalence of acute and chronic prostatitis to be 2.7%.[5] However, it must be stated that the exact prevalence is difficult to ascertain given the variances in diagnostic measures and criteria applied to patient diagnoses by clinicians.

PATIENT VIGNETTE

Matt is a 45-year-old male who is new to your practice and presents to establish care and seek a more urgent evaluation for a new urinary issue. Upon rooming the patient, your medical assistant informs you that, "Matt looks pretty sick" and is running a fever of 101°F, has complaints of chills, and "he looks pretty worn down". She states that his major complaint is dysuria, urinary frequency, weaker urinary stream, urinary dribbling, and pain when having a bowel movement. The patients' history is significant for symptoms that have been present for the past 5 d and Matt is really concerned because he has not felt well enough to engage in sexual activity with his new girlfriend of 1 mo. He states that he really likes this girl and they started the week off celebrating her return from a business trip, but he is fearful she is going to think less of him for not wanting to engage in sexual activity over the last 4 to 5 d. Upon examination you note a patient that is stable, but appears acutely ill. Pertinent physical examination findings reveal that Matt has tenderness in his testicles, and some tenderness of the glans penis. You note generalized abdominal pain, but no definitive findings that warrant emergent evaluation with radiologic imaging. You have a strong differential diagnosis of acute bacterial prostatitis (ABP) when your digital rectal examination (DRE) reveals a soft, boggy, mildly edematous, and acutely tender prostate gland that causes Matt to wince upon palpation.

EPIDEMIOLOGY

The pathogenesis of prostatitis nearly always involves entry of microbes through the urethra whereby microorganisms translocate through the prostatic ducts from the urethra and/or the bladder. In a smaller number of cases, infection is noted from transrectal manipulative procedures, such as a transrectal prostate biopsy or urethral procedures, such as urinary catheterization or cystoscopy.[6–9] Acute prostatitis is also a common presentation in the setting of containment infection of cystitis, urethritis, and other urogenital tract infection, such as epididymitis.[7] Contributory factors such as anatomic and functional anomalies including urethral stricture and intraprostatic reflux infected of urine have been postulated as 2 additional mechanisms of infection.[10] Patients with immunocompromising conditions, such as men with human immunodeficiency virus (HIV), are noted to be diagnosed with lower urinary tract symptoms, including prostatitis, more frequently than men in the general population without a diagnosis of HIV; the exact cause for increased symptomatology is not known at this time.[11]

Similarly, it has long been thought that trauma, dehydration, sexual abstinence, and heavy exercise predispose men to prostatitis, but several well-controlled studies have not found a direct correlation between these causative factors. Risk factors for the development of CBP are also poorly defined in the literature. However, literature does support increased diagnosis of CBP in men who were initially diagnosed with acute prostatitis, men who had procedural manipulation of the urinary tract, men who had a prior diagnosis of diabetes, nicotine addiction, and men who were found on physical examination to have a higher prostate volume.[12] The presence of prostatic stones also appears to have some degree of causation in the increased diagnosis of CBP.[13]

Microorganisms that are responsible for both acute and CBP are synonymous with microbes that are responsible for other urogenital tract infections in men including cystitis, urethritis, and epididymitis. The gram-negative microbe, *Escherichia coli* (*E. coli*), is noted to be the most prevalent offender, followed by *Proteus* species, then *Klebsiella, Enterobacter,* and *Serratia* Enterobacterales, and finally *Pseudomonas aeruginosa.* In a more limited number of cases, gram-positive pathogens of *Staphylococcus aureus, Streptococci,* and *Enterococci* have been isolated. Clinicians should be concerned and begin a workup for a remote or endovascular *Staphylococcal* infection in patients where prostatic fluid cultures *Staphylococcal* prostatitis. *Neisseria gonorrhoeae, Chlamydia trachomatis,* and *Mycoplasma genitalium* have also been implicated as causative organisms responsible for prostatitis in younger male patients who are sexually active and should be considered as the basis for infection in men who also have a diagnosis of urethritis and/or epididymitis or in patients who have immunocompromising conditions, such as men with a diagnosis of HIV.[8,14,15] Finally, the literature cites rare cases where fungal organisms were responsible for acute and chronic prostatitis, but these were observed in patients who had underlying immunosuppression or were actively receiving immunosuppressive therapy,[16–18] **Table 2.**

Table 2	
Pathogens responsible for acute and chronic prostatitis	
Classification	**Pathogens**
Gram negative pathogens	*E. Coli – up to 80% of infections, Proteus, Klebsiella, Enterobacter, Serratia, Klebsiella pneumoniae, Proteus mirabilis, Pseudomonas aeruginosa*
Gram positive pathogens	*Staphylococcus aureus, streptococci, enterococci*
Sexually transmitted pathogens	*Neisseria gonorrhoeae, Chlamydia trachomatis, Mycoplasma genitalium*
Fungal organisms	*Mycoplasma tuberculosis, Candida spp., Coccidioides immitis, Blastomyces dermatitidis, Histoplasma capsulatum*

CLINICAL PRESENTATION

Prostatitis, whether acute or chronic, presents as a clinical syndrome with a variety of urinary symptoms. Patients with acute prostatitis will frequently present with a sepsis clinical picture and symptoms including: malaise, fever, chills, dysuria, urinary frequency, urinary hesitancy, a slower than baseline urinary stream, and may or may not have symptoms or urinary obstruction or urinary retention.[19,20] Patients will most commonly complain of pain in the scrotum, testes, the perineum, the penile body or glans, suprapubic pain, and may have concerns for low back pain. DRE will reveal an intensely tender prostate gland that may be soft, edematous, and boggy or more firm to palpation. Clinicians must take great care when completing a DRE not to massage the prostate as this can induce bacteremia and sepsis.[18]

In somewhat stark contrast is the patient that presents with CBP. A limited number of these patients will also present with the classic host of symptoms that include: dysuria, urinary frequency, urinary urgency, perineal tenderness, and less likely a low grade fever. Some patients will also have complaints of sexual dysfunction, blood noted in their semen, and/or pain with ejaculation.[19,21] These patients often have a prostate examination that is without regard, but it is possible to note prostate enlargement, mild edema, and less frequently prostate nodularity.[19] The examination for patients with chronic prostatitis is quite subtle in nature and some patients are asymptomatic with only persistent or recurrent bacteriuria responsible for their diagnosis.

MEDICAL/PHARMACOLOGIC MANAGEMENT

The selection of an effective treatment for bacterial prostatitis is contingent upon several critical factors, including the classification of the infection as either acute or chronic, patient demographics such as age and associated risk factors including the potential for sexually transmitted infections (STIs).

Treatment should focus on selecting an antimicrobial agent with an appropriate spectrum of activity and sufficient penetration into prostate tissue. Treating prostatitis presents challenges for antibiotic delivery due to the prostate being alkaline with reduced capillary permeability compared to other body tissues. In ABP, significant inflammation increases vascular flow, improving antibiotic penetration and expanding treatment options. Due to the enhanced antibiotic penetration related to increased vascular flow during acute infections, they can usually be treated with shorter treatment durations compared to chronic prostatitis.

Best practices dictate that antimicrobial therapy should be guided by culture and sensitivity results. However, obtaining these for prostatitis may be challenging due to the anatomic location and nature of the infection. Therefore, empiric therapy should be initiated to target organisms commonly associated with ABP, which are gram-negative enteric bacteria including, *E. coli, Klebsiella species, Proteus species, Pseudomonas aeruginosa*, and *Enterobacter* species. *Neisseria gonorrhoeae* and *Chlamydia trachomatis* should be given higher consideration as potential pathogens in men with prostatitis who are under the age of 35 and in men over the age of 35 who report engaging in high-risk sexual activities that increase their susceptibility to STIs.[22,23] Additionally, pathogens such as *E. coli, Klebsiella, Proteus*, and *Enterococcus* species should be suspected as the pathogen in men who engage in sex with men and are the insertive partner during anal intercourse.[24]

For patients with ABP under the age of 35 or those over 35 who report high-risk sexual practices, treatment should include a single dose of ceftriaxone 500 mg intramuscularly (IM) followed by 1 dose of azithromycin 1000 mg or doxycycline 100 mg orally twice daily for 10 to 14 d. This regimen targets *Neisseria gonorrhoeae* and *Chlamydia*

Table 3
Antibiotics used in treatment

Patient Population	Medication	Dosage
High Risk Sexual Practices	Ceftriaxone AND Azithromycin OR Doxycycline	500 mg IM 1000 mg x 1 dose 100 mg PO BID x 10–14 d
No High-Risk Sexual Practice	Ciprofloxacin OR Levofloxacin OR trimethoprim/ sulfamethoxazole (DS)	500 mg PO BID x 10–14 d 500–750 mg PO BID x 10–14 d 800 mg/160 mg PO BID x 10–14 d

trachomatis.[25] Conversely, men with ABP who have a low risk for STIs should receive either ciprofloxacin 500 mg orally twice daily or levofloxacin 500 to 750 mg orally once daily for 10 to 14 d or trimethoprim/sulfamethoxazole (DS) at a dosage of 1 tablet orally twice daily for the same duration. These antibiotics effectively cover *E. coli, Klebsiella species, Proteus species, Pseudomonas aeruginosa,* and *Enterobacter* species.[25] Refer to **Table 3**.

Most patients will experience resolution of their ABP symptoms within 2 w of treatment. However, if symptoms persist beyond this period, further evaluations should be conducted, including repeated complete blood count, urinalysis, and urine and blood cultures. In such cases, the antimicrobial regimen should be extended for an additional 2 w. If patients show no response to therapy or if their symptoms worsen, the possibility of a prostate abscess and the possibility of sepsis must be considered, which should prompt the clinician to consider hospitalization.[25]

The pathogens associated with CBP are similar to those implicated in ABP, with *E. coli* being the most prevalent. The duration of treatment of CBP is typically extended to 4 to 6 w. In cases where a bacterial cause is confirmed or if the initial treatment results in partial but incomplete symptomatic response, a second 4-to-6-w course of antibiotic therapy may be considered.

Fluoroquinolones are the antibiotic of choice for CBP with levofloxacin being preferred over ciprofloxacin due to its higher rate of bacterial clearance.[26,27] DS, azithromycin, fosfomycin, and aminoglycoside antibiotics are considered alternatives to fluoroquinolones in the treatment of CBP in those who have issues with allergy, intolerance, long QT syndrome, and tendonitis.[24,28] Azithromycin should also always be avoided in patients with a history of long QT syndrome to prevent cardiovascular complications.

Supportive therapy for ABP includes the use of antipyretics, analgesics, stool softeners, time off work, bed rest, and increased fluid intake. Additionally, the use of alpha-blockers such as terazosin 5 mg orally once daily may be beneficial. These medications can enhance bladder outflow and reduce the risk of intraprostatic urinary reflux, thereby alleviating some symptoms associated with ABP.[29] Patients with CBP should be referred to and co-managed with an urologist or nurse practitioner (NP) specializing in urology.

EMERGING THERAPIES/EMERGING TREATMENT

Emerging therapies for the treatment of prostatitis, especially CBP, focus on a variety of innovative approaches aimed at alleviating symptoms and improving quality-of-life for patients. Innovative therapies include botulinum toxin injections, interventional techniques, and complimentary therapies among others.

Botulinum toxin is known to cause muscle relaxation by blocking the release of acetylcholine. It can have a positive effect on sensory neurotransmitters and inflammation. While promising, the evidence of using botulinum injections to alleviate the pain associated with CBP is limited, so the application remains off-label use at this time. Further, large, randomized control trials are necessary to support its use in the treatment of CBP.[30]

Interventional therapies including PAE and transurethral microwave thermotherapy (TUMT) are being investigated for their efficacy in treating the pain and urinary symptoms associated with CBP. PAE blocks the flow of blood to areas of the prostate resulting death and necrosis in some areas of the prostate and a desired decrease in prostatic volume and size. It has most commonly been used in the treatment of benign prostatic hyperplasia (BPH) but has shown some improvement in pain related to chronic prostatitis.[31] TUMT uses microwave-induced heat to ablate prostatic tissue. The heat causes a reduction in prostatic volume and is theoretically postulated to result in improved CBP symptoms. TUMT has been approved for use in the treatment of BPH but not currently for CBP as randomized control studies are needed to determine its efficacy.[32]

Complimentary therapies can include pelvic floor rehabilitation (PFR), which is an important and often overlooked therapy for patients with significant pelvic pain or chronic pelvic pain syndrome due to their CBP. PFR can include physiotherapy, biofeedback, local heat application, and the teaching of relaxation exercises. The utilization of certain medications including diazepam, baclofen, or cyclobenzaprine may be helpful when used carefully in conjunction with PFR.[33]

CONTINUITY OF CARE

Continuity of care is critical for the effective management of both acute and CBP. ABP is commonly addressed in primary care settings by NPs and other healthcare providers. In cases where patients do not respond to standard antibiotic therapy and supportive measures, further diagnostic evaluations are essential to rule out serious complications such as prostatic abscess or sepsis, which can be life-threatening and likely require hospitalization. These patients are typically referred to an urologist or NPs specializing in urology for more intensive management.

CBP, on the other hand, often necessitates a more collaborative approach between primary care and urology. Due to the complex and recurrent nature of the condition, successful treatment frequently involves a multidisciplinary team. This team may include urologists, pain management specialists, PFR therapists, sex therapists, and mental health professionals.

Patients, who lack access to a full multidisciplinary team, may benefit from utilizing telemedicine resources and care to improve outcomes and reduce the risk of complications.

SUMMARY

In summary, the effective management of acute and CBP hinges on timely diagnosis, appropriate antimicrobial therapy, and supportive care. ABP often responds well to antibiotics, but more complex or resistant cases may require further evaluation and specialist involvement to avoid complications like abscess or sepsis. CBP poses a greater challenge due to its recurrent nature and may benefit from a multidisciplinary approach involving urology, pain management, and pelvic floor therapy. Emerging treatments and complementary therapies offer additional hope for symptom relief, while continuity of care, including telemedicine options, plays a crucial role in long-term patient outcomes.

CLINICS CARE POINTS

- Treatment of prostatitis is nuanced by an intracity of syndromes that each require specific treatment, see Table 1.

- Acute prostatitis is common in the setting of containment infection of cystitis, urethritis, and other urogenital tract infection, such as epididymitis.

- Patients with immunocompromising conditions, such as men with HIV, are noted to be diagnosed with lower urinary tract symptoms, including prostatitis, more frequently than men in the general population.

- Trauma, dehydration, sexual abstinence, and heavy exercise have long been thought to predispose men to prostatitis, but several well-controlled studies have not found a direct correlation between these causative factors.

- Patients with acute prostatitis will frequently present with a sepsis clinical picture and symptoms including: malaise, fever, chills, dysuria, urinary frequency, urinary hesitancy, a slower than baseline urinary stream, and may or may not have symptoms or urinary obstruction or urinary retention.

- Men who report high-risk sexual practices, treatment should include a single dose of ceftriaxone 500 mg IM followed by 1 dose of azithromycin 1000 mg or doxycycline 100 mg orally twice daily for 10 to 14 d. This regimen targets *Neisseria gonorrhoeae* and *Chlamydia trachomatis*.

- Men with ABP who have a low risk for STIs should receive ciprofloxacin, levofloxacin, or DS for 10 to 14 d.

- Patient who show no response to therapy or have symptoms that worsen should prompt the NP to consider the possibility of a prostate abscess, which can lead to sepsis.

- In patients who show partial improvement, but not resolution of symptoms with initial antibiotic therapy, a second 4-to-6-w course of antibiotic therapy should be considered.

- The antibiotic of choice for CBP are fluoroquinolones, with levofloxacin having a higher preference over ciprofloxacin due its higher rate of bacterial clearance

- Non-pharmaceutical therapies can include: PFR, physiotherapy, biofeedback, local heat application, and the teaching of relaxation exercises.

- Additional pharmaceutical therapies can include: diazepam, baclofen, or cyclobenzaprine when used carefully in conjunction with PFR.

DISCLOSURES

The authors have nothing to disclose.

REFERENCES

1. Su ZT, Zenilman JM, Sfanos KS, et al. Management of chronic bacterial prostatitis. Curr Urol Rep 2020;21:1–8.
2. Krieger JN, Nyberg Jr L, Nickel JC. NIH consensus definition and classification of prostatitis. JAMA 1999;282(3):236–7.
3. Potts J, Payne RE. Prostatitis: infection, neuromuscular disorder, or pain syndrome? Proper patient classification is key. Cleve Clin J Med 2007;74(3):S63.
4. Pontari MA, Joyce GF, Wise M, et al, Urologic Diseases in America Project. Urologic diseases in America project. Prostatitis. J Urol 2007;177(6):2050–7.
5. Gasperi M, Krieger JN, Panizzon MS, et al. Genetic and environmental influences on urinary conditions in men: a classical twin study. Urology 2019;129:54–9.

6. Johnson JR, Kuskowski MA, Gajewski A, et al. Extended virulence genotypes and phylogenetic background of Escherichia coli isolates from patients with cystitis, pyelonephritis, or prostatitis. J Infect Dis 2005;191(1):46–50.

7. Krieger JN, Dobrindt U, Riley DE, et al. Acute Escherichia coli prostatitis in previously health young men: bacterial virulence factors, antimicrobial resistance, and clinical outcomes. Urology 2011;77(6):1420–5.

8. Kim SH, Ha US, Yoon BI, et al. Microbiological and clinical characteristics in acute bacterial prostatitis according to lower urinary tract manipulation procedure. J Infect Chemother 2014;20(1):38–42.

9. Ramakrishnan K, Salinas RC. Prostatitis: acute and chronic. Prim Care Clin Off Pract 2010;37(3):547–63.

10. Karlovsky ME, Pontari MA. Theories of prostatitis etiology. Curr Urol Rep 2002; 3(4):307–12.

11. Breyer BN, Van Den Eeden SK, Horberg MA, et al. HIV status is an independent risk factor for reporting lower urinary tract symptoms. J Urol 2011;185(5):1710–5.

12. Yoon BI, Kim S, Han DS, et al. Acute bacterial prostatitis: how to prevent and manage chronic infection? J Infect Chemother 2012;18(4):444–50.

13. Zhao WP, Li YT, Chen J, et al. Prostatic calculi influence the antimicrobial efficacy in men with chronic bacterial prostatitis. Asian J Androl 2012;14(5):715.

14. Nagy V, Kubej D. Acute bacterial prostatitis in humans: current microbiological spectrum, sensitivity to antibiotics and clinical findings. Urol Int 2012;89(4):445–50.

15. Workowski KA, Bachmann LH, Chan PA, et al. Sexually transmitted infections treatment guidelines, 2021. MMWR. Recommendations and Reports 2021;70.

16. Humphrey PA. Fungal prostatitis caused by coccidioides. J Urol 2014;191(1): 215–6.

17. Larsen RA, Bozzette S, McCutchan JA, et al, California Collaborative Treatment Group. Persistent Cryptococcus neoformans infection of the prostate after successful treatment of meningitis. Ann Intern Med 1989;111(2):125–8.

18. Kranz J, Bartoletti R, Bruyère F, et al. European association of urology guidelines on urological infections: summary of the 2024 guidelines. Eur Urol 2024;86(1): 27–41.

19. Pirola GM, Verdacchi T, Rosadi S, et al. Chronic prostatitis: current treatment options. Res Rep Urol 2019;4:165–74.

20. Coker TJ, Dierfeldt DM. Acute bacterial prostatitis: diagnosis and management. Am Fam Physician 2016;93(2):114–20.

21. Müller A, Mulhall JP. Sexual dysfunction in the patient with prostatitis. Curr Opin Urol 2005;15(6):404–9.

22. Coker TJ, Dierfeldt DM. Acute bacterial prostatitis: diagnosis and management. Am Fam Physician 2016;93(2):114–20.

23. Xiong S, Liu X, Deng W, et al. Pharmacological interventions for bacterial prostatitis. Front Pharmacol 2020;11:504.

24. Nickel JC, Dow G. Prostatitis: acute and chronic bacterial prostatitis and chronic pelvic pain syndrome. In: Mulhall JL, Traish LM, Perito AJ, editors. Current clinical urology. United States: Springer; 2016. p. 59–79.

25. Xiong S, Liu X, Deng W, et al. Pharmacological interventions for bacterial prostatitis. Front Pharmacol 2020;11:504. PMID: 32425775; PMCID: PMC7203426.

26. Zhang ZC, Jin FS, Liu DM, et al. Safety and efficacy of levofloxacin versus ciprofloxacin for the treatment of chronic bacterial prostatitis in Chinese patients. Asian J Androl 2012;14(6):870–4.

27. Perletti G, Marras E, Wagenlehner FM, et al. Antimicrobial therapy for chronic bacterial prostatitis. Cochrane Database Syst Rev 2013;2013(8):CD009071.

28. Cunha BA, Gran A, Raza M. Persistent extended-spectrum β-lactamase-positive Escherichia coli chronic prostatitis successfully treated with a combination of fosfomycin and doxycycline. Int J Antimicrob Agents 2015;45(4):427–9.

29. Barbalias GA, Nikiforidis G, Liatsikos EN. Alpha-blockers for the treatment of chronic prostatitis in combination with antibiotics. J Urol 1998;159(3):883–7.

30. Chen CH, Tyagi P, Chuang YC. Promise and the pharmacological mechanism of botulinum toxin A in chronic prostatitis syndrome. Toxins (Basel) 2019;11(10):586. PMID: 31614473; PMCID: PMC6832516.

31. Parikh N, Keshishian E, Sharma A, et al. Prostatic artery embolization is safe and effective for medically recalcitrant radiation-induced prostatitis. Adv Radiat Oncol 2020;5(5):905–9. PMID: 33083652; PMCID: PMC7557125.

32. Franco JV, Garegnani L, Escobar Liquitay CM, et al. Transurethral microwave thermotherapy for the treatment of lower urinary tract symptoms in men with benign prostatic hyperplasia. Cochrane Database Syst Rev 2021;6(6):CD004135. PMID: 34180047; PMCID: PMC8236484.

33. Doiron RC, Nickel JC. Management of chronic prostatitis/chronic pelvic pain syndrome. Can Urol Assoc J 2018;12(6 Suppl 3):S161–3. PMID: 29875042; PMCID: PMC6040620.

Moving?

Make sure your subscription moves with you!

To notify us of your new address, find your **Clinics Account Number** (located on your mailing label above your name), and contact customer service at:

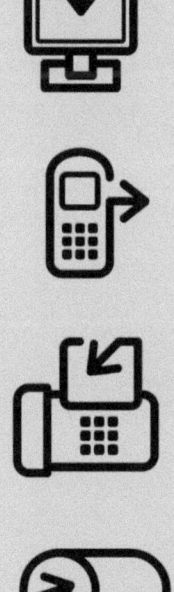

Email: journalscustomerservice-usa@elsevier.com

800-654-2452 (subscribers in the U.S. & Canada)
314-447-8871 (subscribers outside of the U.S. & Canada)

Fax number: 314-447-8029

Elsevier Health Sciences Division
Subscription Customer Service
3251 Riverport Lane
Maryland Heights, MO 63043

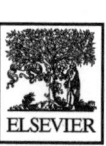

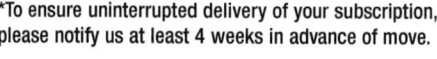
*To ensure uninterrupted delivery of your subscription, please notify us at least 4 weeks in advance of move.